Succeeding on your Nursing Placement

Succeeding on your Nursing Placement

SUPERVISION, LEARNING AND ASSESSMENT FOR NURSING STUDENTS

Edited by

Ian Peate OBE FRCN
Editor in Chief British Journal of Nursing
Visiting Professor St Georges University of
London and Kingston University London;
Visiting Professor Northumbria University;
Professorial Fellow Roehampton University;
Visiting Senior Clinical Fellow University
of Hertfordshire, UK

WILEY Blackwell

Registered Offices
John Wiley & Sons, Inc., 111 River Street, Hoboken, NJ 07030, USA
John Wiley & Sons Ltd, The Atrium, Southern Gate, Chichester, West Sussex, PO19 8SQ, UK

For details of our global editorial offices, customer services, and more information about Wiley products visit us at www.wiley.com.

Wiley also publishes its books in a variety of electronic formats and by print-on-demand. Some content that appears in standard print versions of this book may not be available in other formats.

Library of Congress Cataloging-in-Publication Data applied for:
[PB ISBN: 9781119819660]

Cover Design: Wiley
Cover Image: © Reza Estakhrian/Getty Images, FS Productions/Getty Images

Set in 10/12pt STIXTwoText by Straive, Pondicherry, India
Printed and bound by CPI Group (UK) Ltd, Croydon, CR0 4YY

C9781119819660_140823

BRIEF CONTENTS

CONTENTS

4 Equality and diversity needs 72

Sue Jackson, Claire Camara, and Peta Jane Greaves

5 Learning in practice 94

Lucy Tyler and Paulette Ragan

6 Getting ready for practice 119

Mariama Seray-Wurie

9 The practice assessment document 183

Jane Fish and Kathy Wilson

10 Receiving feedback and feedforward 214

Siobhan McGuckin

11 The student as a teacher   238

12 Lifelong learning 269

CONTRIBUTORS

Sebastian Birch
RMN, FHEA
Sebastian is a senior clinical nurse specialist working in a child and adolescent mental health services team in South-West London as the risk and self-harm lead. He is adept at delivering psychosocial interventions (based on dialectical behavioural therapy and mentalisation-based therapy). He has also been a senior lecturer at Roehampton University and continues to work as a visiting lecturer. He works to bring philosophical concepts into nursing to deepen our understanding of care. He has studied for a masters in continental philosophy, which he uses to critique and expand the foundations of care.

Claire Camara
RN
Claire is a lecturer in children and young people's nursing at Northumbria University. She is currently undertaking a PhD aiming to understand the lived experience of young people who have a chronic illness and are currently taking part in a clinical trial. Previously, Claire worked as a paediatric research nurse supporting children, young people and their families throughout their research journey. Claire has also cared for patients and their families in paediatric oncology, forensic units and in-patient eating disorders. Her research interests include the lived experiences of children and young people, the student experience, and end of life care provision. Claire is also co-lead of the health and life sciences student equality, diversity and inclusion group at Northumbria University and is working with students on different initiatives within that group.

Luke Cox
RN, BSc (Hons), PGDE, FHEA
Luke qualified as a nurse in 2005 and has experience in cardiology and emergency department settings. He has worked as a clinical educator,

focusing on using simulation as a teaching methodology. He is currently a senior lecturer in clinical skills and simulation at the University of Roehampton.

Jane Fish
RN, RCNT, RNT, DipN (Lond), DipN Ed (Lond), MBA

Jane has her own successful consultancy business in management, education and training. Jane started nursing in 1979 and undertook three years of student nurse training at the Thomas Guy School of Nursing in London. She completed post-registration courses in intensive care and care of the elderly and was a ward sister at Guy's Hospital in medicine and rehabilitation of the elderly. Moving into nurse education in 1988, she studied at the Institute of Advanced Nurse Education at the Royal College of Nursing in 1989 and 1991, completing the Diploma in Nurse Education with distinction. In 1994, Jane graduated from the Open Business School with a Master's in Business Administration. Since 1993, Jane has established her consultancy business. She has collaborated with multiple stakeholders in NHS trusts, universities, the Department of Health, CapitalNurse and Health Education England, working at a national, regional and local level. Jane has extensive project management experience and was project manager on the first Pan London Practice Assessment Document (PLPAD) project for pre-registration nursing students in 2013 and project managed the second PLPAD from 2017 to 2019 to prepare future nurses, with the document being used by most universities across England.

Peta Jane Greaves
RGN, PhD

Jane Greaves is an associate professor in the Faculty of Health and Life Sciences at the University of Northumbria, where she has worked for 14 years. She is a registered nurse with 13 years' experience of working in critical care. Subsequently, she worked for six years as a lecturer practitioner promoting interprofessional education in the context of patient deterioration, particularly between doctors and nurses, when managing acute deterioration. Jane has continued to pursue interests in interprofessional education and its role in patient safety. In her doctoral thesis, she studied the use of early warning scores. Jane is a trustee and honorary treasurer of the National Confidential Enquiry into Patient Outcome and Death. More recently, she has investigated the application of early warning scores in the community and learning disability sectors.

Sue Jackson
PhD RNT FHEA
Sue Jackson is an associate professor in adult nursing at Northumbria University, Newcastle upon Tyne. She is a registered nurse with 37 years working within clinical nursing, healthcare research and nurse education. Her doctoral thesis examined 'Student nurse professionalism: repertoires and discourses used by university students and their lecturers'. This work explores the student journey to professional socialisation through the language they use. Her research interests aim to enhance the student's experience in both the academic and clinical setting. As departmental director for equality, diversity and inclusion, Sue is committed to ensuring that students from minority and widening participation groups have a voice at all stages of their education journey.

Catherine Jones
RN, BA (Hons), DipHE (Nurs), PGCE Healthcare
Professionals, FHEA
Catherine's nursing career began as a staff nurse in a busy London teaching hospital in 1997. After gaining some useful experience, she joined the critical care team and gained specialist qualifications in intensive care nursing in 2003. Later, Catherine was fortunate to be able to work as a junior sister on a general surgery ward and senior staff nurse in an intensive care setting. Supporting students in practice was integral to her nursing practice throughout these years and in 2014 Catherine became practice educator and team leader on the general intensive care unit. Catherine joined the team at the University of Roehampton in August 2020 as a senior lecturer in nurse education and enjoys teaching pre-registration nursing students. Her interests include critical care, non-technical skills, simulation, workforce development and lifelong learning.

Serena Khoury
Serena is a third-year student mental health nurse and programme representative for the same course at the University of Roehampton. She has completed placement in a plethora of mental health services during her time at Roehampton, including the Priory, Change Grow Live and Barnes Hospital. She is interested in the exploration of trauma in childhood and how that affects people in adulthood. When she graduates, she would like to work in eating disorder services for adults and hopes to open a mental health clinic in West Africa one day.

Kim Lewin
RN, MSc, Specialist Practitioner, DipHE (Nursing),
Independent and Supplementary Prescriber, FHEA, Queen's
Nurse
In her nursing career, Kim has worked in a variety of roles including those of practice nurse, nurse practitioner, community matron, specialist nurse and lead for case management. She has worked across acute hospital care, general practice and community settings. After spending many years supporting and assessing students in clinical practice, she moved into the role of senior lecturer in nurse education at the University of Roehampton in 2020, where she teaches BSc adult and mental health students and MSc dual field (adult/mental health) students. Her professional interests include pharmacology, community nursing, complex case management and lifelong learning.

Ashley Luchmun
RN, DN, MA Ed, PG Dip
Ashley began his nursing journey in 2003 registering with the Nursing and Midwifery Council in 2006. He has worked exclusively in community nursing in different roles: community staff nurse, district nurse team manager, community matron and community specialist respiratory nurse. Ashley has always had an inclination for education and joined nursing higher education in 2014. She has since worked in three London universities, teaching mainly on pre-registration and other health care associated programmes. His areas of interest are public health, management of long-term conditions and evidence-based practice. His research area is the use of virtual reality and technology in health education.

Siobhan McGuckin
RGN, MSc, FHEA
Siobhan qualified in 1986 in Belfast, Northern Ireland, and initially worked in the general intensive care unit at the Mater Infirmorum Hospital in Belfast. She then spent time in a nursing home in Rochdale, Lancashire, caring for young disabled patients and patients with multiple sclerosis. Siobhan moved to London, where she commenced her cancer nursing career, especially within haematology. She was the clinical nurse specialist for patients with rare blood disorders: thrombotic microangiopathies at University College Hospital, London. Siobhan has always been involved with teaching and eventually moved into undergraduate nurse education in University College Hospital, London, as a practice educator. From here, she moved into her first academic

position at the University of Roehampton in January 2021. Siobhan's key areas of interest are haematology, person-centred care and preventing and managing deterioration.

Ian Peate
OBE, FRCN
Ian is Editor in Chief British Journal of Nursing, Visiting Professor St Georges University, University of London, and Kingston University, London, Visiting Professor Northumbria University, Professorial Fellow University of Roehampton, Visiting Senior Clinical Fellow University Hertfordshire. He has worked in nurse education since 1989. His key areas of interest are nursing practice and theory. Ian has published widely. Ian was awarded an OBE in the Queen's 90th Birthday Honours List for his services to nursing and nurse education and was granted a fellowship from the Royal College of Nursing in 2017.

Paulette Ragan
RN, BA (Hons), PGCE (Lond)
Paulette started out as an auxiliary nurse in elderly care and commenced training at Westminster Hospital, London, in 1990. Her nursing career has spanned over 30 years of clinical practice in numerous settings in London, Bristol and across Australia. She has worked as a clinical nurse specialist in homelessness and as a community-based practice development nurse as well as a community practice educator. She currently works as a senior lecturer in adult nursing in the nursing and life sciences department at the University of Roehampton Croydon Campus. Her areas of specific interest are public health, marginalised groups, pharmacology and professionalism.

Jo Rixon
RGN, MA Ed, SFHEA
Jo commenced her career in 1986, training at the Hammersmith Hospital School of Nursing. Her clinical career spanned a number of years, primarily remaining within North West London, with a focus on surgical and intensive care nursing. A move to practice development, supporting pre-registration learners within clinical practice, preceded a subsequent move to nurse education in 2006. Jo's initial focus was adult nursing until 2015 when she became head of practice learning and, in 2021, head of nursing. Jo has particular interests in widening participation and supporting career progression, management and leadership and practice learning.

Scott Rodden
RN, BSc (Hons), PGCLT, FHEA
Scott has worked as a staff nurse in cardiology and neurosurgery and has since moved into nurse education. He moved into nurse education in 2021 taking up a nurse lecturer post at BPP University and has since moved to the University of Roehampton as a lecturer in adult nursing. Scott is currently undertaking his master's degree in education, policy and society at Kings College London. His key areas of interest are social justice in nursing and nurse education.

Mariama Seray-Wurie
RN(A), MA, SFHEA
Mariama is head of practice learning, University of Roehampton, responsible for strategic and operational oversight of practice learning, ensuring effective practice learning processes for the nursing programme that meet the university and regulatory body requirements. She became a registered nurse in 1989 and her clinical background was in infectious diseases and haematology. She moved into higher education in 2000, starting her career in nurse education as a clinical skills facilitator. Mariama has been a lecturer at the University of West London, a senior lecturer for adult nursing and a director of programmes at Middlesex University. She graduated with an MA in learning and teaching in healthcare in 2005. Mariama's teaching focus is mainly with pre-registration nursing curriculum development and programme management, simulated practice learning and international exchanges in nursing.

Lucy Tyler
RN, MSc, FHEA
Lucy has been a qualified nurse since 2004. Her clinical career has been spent mainly in neurology and emergency nursing. She has always had a passion for facilitating the learning of others either in clinical practice or in recent years within higher education, where she has been involved in a variety of education innovations in undergraduate nursing education. Lucy has a keen interest in clinical skills and simulation-based education, integrating mental and physical health and interprofessional learning within nurse education.

Laura Wasey
Laura is a student nurse.

Kathy Wilson
RN, PhD (Professional Studies), Dip N, PGCHE
Kathy is director of professional practice at Middlesex University, London. She started her nursing career in 1983. Kathy has spent much of her academic career in roles that have focused on practice learning and assessment as this is where her passion lies. As chair of the Pan London Practice Learning Group (PLPLG), Kathy has overseen the development of the second Pan London Practice Assessment Document (PAD), with the support of a project manager, funded by Health Education England and a large group of pan-London HEI and practice partner colleagues. This work led to the creation of a range of online resources to support the development of practice assessors and practice supervisors and these e-modules can be accessed via the PLPLG website. Following the successful implementation of the PAD, Kathy secured further funding to support the development of an electronic PAD, which is transforming the student and supervisor/assessor experience across London. She chairs the Pan London ePAD steering group.

PREFACE

Succeeding on your Nursing Placement helps students of nursing and other health and social care students understand the principles required to learn effectively and make the most out of the learning experience in various health and care settings. The contributors are academics and clinicians with an ability to draw on many years' experience in nursing practice and nurse education.

Pre-registration nursing students and trainee nursing associates are required by the Nursing and Midwifery Council (NMC) to achieve a minimum number of practice hours during their programme of study. The NMC introduced new education standards in 2018 these new standards (also known as the Future Nurse Standards; NMC 2018a) reflect the scope and requirements of contemporary nursing practice. For the first time, the NMC also produced Standards of Proficiency for Nursing Associates (NMC 2018b). These standards impact nursing students, nurse apprenticeships and trainee nursing associates. The standards also affect those nurses who wish to return to practice, all registered nurses, nursing associates, higher education institutions such as universities, and practice placement providers.

With the introduction of the new NMC education standards, the way in which practice-based learning is assessed and delivered has also changed. Students are still required to undertake a prescribed number of practice-based learning hours before they can be registered with the NMC. There has been a significant change to practice-based learning. Mentors and sign-off mentors have now been replaced with practice supervisors, practice assessors and academic assessors. The Standards for Student Supervision and Assessment were also introduced in 2018 (NMC 2018c). Nurse education, as noted, has and is changing dramatically, as students, practitioners and academics respond to challenges faced locally, nationally and internationally. Over the past few years there has been significant disruption to the provision of nurse education. The COVID-19 pandemic has seen care provision and nurse education adapt, with the art and science of caring remaining central to all that is taught.

We acknowledge, from the outset, that there are many names used in the literature to describe those who would share their illness experience with students of nursing, including patients, clients, consumers, stakeholders, service users, patient educators, patient instructors, clinical teaching associates, supervisors and mentors. For the sake of clarity and conciseness, we have chosen to use the term 'patient' to denote those with illness experience and their caregivers who may participate in health profession education. We accept the understanding that the history and etymology of the word 'patient' can be challenging, and that the term can be associated with passivity and being acted upon.

Succeeding on your Nursing Placement gives much consideration to the Standards for Student Supervision and Assessment (NMC 2018c), which are applicable to all students, and how they are used in practice settings. Learning in practice is a fundamental part of every student's formal education, often presenting challenges to all who are involved in practice-based learning. Some students report that they encounter a range of difficulties as they try to fit into the practice environment, for a number of reasons. As a result, they must be prepared for their role through the development of appropriate skills as they learn in practice.

All students who undertake a nursing programme must complete practice placements. These placement hours are an essential requirement for registration. Practice placements can cause students stress and this can compromise learning. Thorough preparation by the student and an understanding of the myriad of opportunities that are available in the practice learning environment accompanying a placement can reduce anxiety and enhance the learning experience, which will ultimately result in better, safer patient care.

A student's exposure to the practice learning environment is one of the most important factors affecting the teaching and learning process in health and care settings. Helping students to navigate the sometimes complex learning environments to which they are exposed could improve practice education and also reduce the rates of student attrition.

The key issues that students are likely to face during the practice learning experience are the focus of this text. *Succeeding on your Nursing Placement* is arranged over 12 chapters. The text offers support and advice to encourage students to get the most out of the practice-based placement. The chapters concentrate on helping students as they engage in their practice placements, encouraging them to think about their part in the process and their obligations, as well as the roles and responsibilities of others (NMC 2018d). They are urged to explore what they bring to the placement and what they can expect from the learning experiences. There is an emphasis on acknowledging and recognising one's own responsibilities as well as understanding the responsibilities of the higher education institutions (universities) and the various practice-based partners. The text includes an explanation about how practice-based learning is organised and why; putting the pieces of the jigsaw together. Understanding these issues may help the reader to enjoy a better learning experience.

Our aim is to the engage the reader with a range of interactive activities, so students are able to understand and apply the knowledge to their practice. Where appropriate, there are a number of interactive activities to encourage the reader to take stock and carry out a variety of activities. *Succeeding on your Nursing Placement* adopts a practical approach and where relevant practice exercises are incorporated encouraging students to apply what they are reading to the practice placement experience (wherever this may be). To enhance understanding, the chapters have several summary sections interspaced, enabling the reader to digest the bite-sized discussions. Each chapter begins with an aim and learning outcomes, permitting the reader to contextualise and concentrate on the chapter content.

Succeeding on your Nursing Placement has the potential to help students to seek out and create learning opportunities located within the care environment, and to develop skills related to practice learning, which can help them to reach proficiency and gain confidence. This book is, more than anything else, a practical guide for students who wish to develop skills for learning when in practice placements.

We hope that students will find the content useful as they engage with and in the amazing world of nursing and health care. Nurse education and nursing practice are constantly changing and evolving to meet a multitude of changes and developments, students play a key part in those changes and we wish them much success as they undertake their nursing programmes.

References

Nursing and Midwifery Council (2018a) Future Nurse: Standards of Proficiency for Registered Nurses. https://www.nmc.org.uk/globalassets/sitedocuments/education-standards/future-nurse-proficiencies.pdf (accessed September 2022).

Nursing and Midwifery Council (2018b). Standards of Proficiency for Nursing Associates. https://www.nmc.org.uk/globalassets/sitedocuments/education-standards/nursing-associates-proficiency-standards.pdf (accessed September 2022).

Nursing and Midwifery Council (2018c). Realising Professionalism: Standards for Education and Training. Part 2: Standards for Student Supervision and Assessment. https://www.nmc.org.uk/globalassets/sitedocuments/education-standards/student-supervision-assessment.pdf (accessed September 2022).

Nursing and Midwifery Council (2018d). Standards for Pre-registration Nursing Education. https://www.nmc.org.uk/Programme-standards-nursing (accessed December 2020).

ACKNOWLEDGEMENTS

I would like to thank my partner, Jussi Lahtinen, for his constant support. I also owe recognition to the chapter contributors and students who, despite tumultuous times, supported me in their contributions to the text – thank you all.

CHAPTER 1

Your course, your programme of study

Ian Peate and Scott Rodden

AIM

This chapter provides the reader with insight into how healthcare programmes of study (nursing) are devised and developed, together with regulatory requirements that must be met.

LEARNING OUTCOMES

Having read this chapter, the reader will:

1. Be able to outline the role and function of the Nursing and Midwifery Council.
2. Understand how a programme of study is constructed.
3. Have an awareness of the essential requirements that are associated with a Nursing and Midwifery Council approved programme.
4. Be able to describe the purpose of regulation and the Nursing and Midwifery Council's professional register.

Succeeding on your Nursing Placement: Supervision, Learning and Assessment for Nursing Students, First Edition. Edited by Ian Peate.
© 2024 John Wiley & Sons Ltd. Published 2024 by John Wiley & Sons Ltd.

Introduction

You have enrolled on an educational programme that will prepare you to become a member of a profession that is respected by people around the globe, and which brings with it great privilege and responsibility. As a student, be proud of the profession you are preparing to enter. Throughout your programme of study, aim to uphold the values and standards that have made the UK's nurses so well regarded around the world. It is crucial that, even as a student, you conduct yourself professionally at all times so as to defend the trust that the public places in our profession. Throughout your programme, you will be learning about the behaviour and conduct that the public expects from nurses. On more than one occasion, you will be assessed on the knowledge, skills and behaviours required to become a registered nurse.

In your practice placement (your placement experience), your knowledge, skills, and behaviours are assessed against the personal and professional conduct expected of you as a nursing student to determine whether, after completion of your programme, you will be deemed fit to practice. You will be working towards the standards enshrined in the Code (NMC 2018a) during your pre-registration programme, so it is important that you are aware of and understand these standards, these benchmarks.

The Nursing and Midwifery Council

In the UK, nursing is one of two professions regulated by the Nursing and Midwifery Council (NMC), the other is midwifery. The regulation of nurses and midwives by statute has been in place for over 100 years. This chapter focuses predominantly on nurses. There are other health and social care professions that are also regulated by law; for example, paramedics and operating department practitioners are regulated by the Health and Care Professions Council (HCPC).

Complete this activity now

How many health and care professions does the HCPC regulate? Make a list of them:

It is important that future generations of nurses have an understanding of how nursing as a profession and other health and social care professions have developed and how we have been brought to this point in our evolution as we continue to move forward. Locally, nationally and internationally, we need nurses who practise to the highest of standards, providing patient care that is safe, effective, dynamic and responsive to the changing needs of individuals, communities and nations; this is the hallmark of our profession.

Established by Parliament and with a UK-wide remit, the NMC was formed under the Nursing and Midwifery Order 2001. As the statutory regulator for over 700 000 nurses, nursing associates and midwives (NMC 2022a,b,c), the NMC's core function is to protect the public by setting standards of practice for the professions and to ensure that standards are maintained. Those nurses, nursing associates and midwives whose name appears on the professional register are known collectively as registrants.

The Code

The Code (NMC 2018a) clearly sets out to registrants the professional standards that are required of them as they undertake their professional responsibilities. Although students are not registered with the NMC, it is expected that they keep to the principles expressed within the Code. All registrants must act in line with the Code, whether they are providing direct care to individuals, groups or communities or bringing their professional knowledge to impact on nursing practice in other roles, for example, leadership, education, or research.

Protection of the public is the key concern of the NMC. The NMC's duties to society are to serve and protect, and this is done by:

- Maintaining a register that lists all nurses, nursing associates, and midwives.
- Setting standards and guidelines for nursing and midwifery education, practice and conduct (this also includes nursing associates).
- Ensuring quality assurance related to nursing and midwifery education.
- Considering allegations of misconduct or unfitness to practise as a result of registrant's ill health.

Within the Code is a series of statements that, when considered together, represent what good nursing practice should look like. With the interests of patients and service users paramount, care should be safe and effective and the actions of the nurse should promote trust through professionalism. There are four themes in the Code that describe what nurses are expected to do:

- prioritise people
- practise effectively
- preserve safety, and
- promote professionalism and trust.

Prioritise people

You are required to put the interests of those people who are using or needing nursing services first. You have to ensure that their care and safety is your main concern and that dignity is preserved and their needs are acknowledged, assessed and responded to. Those who are recipients of care are to be treated with respect, ensuring that their rights are defended and that if there are any discriminatory attitudes and behaviours directed towards those receiving care, they are challenged.

Practise effectively

When practising in an effective manner, you will assess needs and deliver or advise on treatment or offer help (this also includes preventative or rehabilitative care) without too much delay and to the best of your abilities and on the foundation of the best available evidence and best practice. You must communicate in an effective manner, ensuring that you keep clear and accurate records and sharing your skills, knowledge and experience where this is appropriate. You must reflect and act on any feedback that you receive with the intention of improving your practice.

Try this on placement

Within your practice assessment document there is opportunity for patients/service users/carers/relatives to provide feedback:

With the Code uppermost in your mind, how can you use the feedback provided to help you improve your practice?

Patient/service user/carer feedback form

Practice supervisors/practice assessors should obtain consent from patients/service users/carers who can if they wish decline to participate. We would very much like to hear your views about the way the student has supported your need. The feedback you provide will not change the way you are cared for; it will help to develop the student's learning.

Tick if you are:	The Patient/Service User ☐		Carer/Relative ☐		
How happy were you with the way the student...	Very Happy	Happy	Unsure	Unhappy	Very Unhappy
...cared for you?	◯	◯	◯	◯	◯
...listened to you?	◯	◯	◯	◯	◯
...understood the way you felt?	◯	◯	◯	◯	◯
...talked to you?	◯	◯	◯	◯	◯
...demonstrated respect towards you?	◯	◯	◯	◯	◯

What did the student do well?

What could the student have done differently?

Practice supervisor/assessor:
Name: Signature: Date:
Student's Name: Signature: Date:

Preserve safety

There is a requirement in the Code to keep the public and patients safe from harm. As a registered practitioner you must work within the limits of your competence, using your professional 'duty of candour', raising concerns immediately whenever you come across any situation that will put patients or public safety at risk and you take necessary action to deal with any concerns where appropriate. These are the foundations of patient safety and, as a student, you also have a role to play in maintaining safety.

Write here

What do you think might be the possible reasons for lapses in safety? Can you list them, thinking about human and material issues that could lead to a breach in safety?

Human error	Material issues
Both	

Promote professionalism and trust

At all times you must uphold the reputation of your profession, displaying a personal commitment to the standards of practice and behaviour that are laid out in the Code. You should be a model of integrity and leadership, so others can aspire to these qualities. When you display commitment, integrity and leadership, this often leads to trust and confidence in the profession from patients, those who are receiving care, other health and care professionals as well as the public.

Green flag
The fundamentals of care

The fundamentals of care cover the essential aspects of caring for a patient. They include but are not limited to nutrition, hydration, bladder, and bowel care, physical handling, and making sure that those people receiving care are kept in clean and hygienic conditions. Furthermore, you must ensure that those receiving care have adequate access to nutrition and hydration, and you must make sure that you offer and provide assistance to those people who cannot feed themselves or drink fluids unaided.

The duty of candour requires nurses to be open and honest with colleagues, patients and healthcare regulators when things go wrong. All healthcare professionals must be open and honest with patients when something goes wrong with their treatment or care which causes, or has the potential to cause, harm, or distress (General Medical Council et al. 2014). You must raise concerns immediately if you are aware of a threat to the safety of a patient or a danger to public protection.

In an emergency situation, as a registered nurse, you have a professional duty to take action. This action may need to be taken even when a nurse is off-duty; the nurse must only act within the limits of their competence. The nurse must arrange, wherever possible, for emergency care to be accessed and provided promptly, taking account of their own safety, the safety of others and the availability of other options for providing care.

Using social media

The NMC has provided guidance on the use of social media which is underpinned by the Code (NMC 2019). Social media should be used responsibly and aligned to NMC guidance as well as any guidance issued by your university or employer.

When social media (e.g. social networking sites) is used in a responsible and appropriate way it provides a number of benefits for nurses and students. It can be used to build and maintain professional relationships, to create or access nursing support networks to enable the discussion of specific issues, interests, research, and clinical experiences with other healthcare professionals locally, nationally, and internationally. It should be noted that the principles that have been outlined in the NMC's guidance can also generally be applied to other forms of online communication; for example:

- personal websites and blogs
- discussion boards
- general content shared online, including text, photographs, images, video, and audio files.

Go online

Access the Code online: www.nmc.org.uk/standards/code. Within the Code there are a number of statements that can be applied to the use of social media. Consider the four components taken from the Code and make notes on the implication they have for you and for the people to whom you offer care to specifically related to the use of social media.

Paragraph	Component	Your notes
1.1	Treat people with kindness, respect and compassion.	
5	As a nurse, midwife or nursing associate, you owe a duty of confidentiality to all those who are receiving care.	
20.6	Stay objective and have clear professional boundaries at all times with people in your care (including those who have been in your care in the past), their families and carers.	
20.10	Use all forms of spoken, written, and digital communication (including social media and networking sites) responsibly.	

McGrath et al. (2019) note that the use of online social media among students is popular, with some creating online platforms for peer support and influence. Health and social care students have to be aware of the potential risks related to how they share information and communicate online. The risks can include misconduct investigations and may conclude in exclusion from studies, resulting in the student being prevented from joining the professional register (Box 1.1).

Box 1.1 | How to use social media responsibly

- Familiarise yourself with how individual social media applications work and be clear about their advantages and disadvantages.
- Think before you post; it is important to realise that even the strictest privacy settings have limitations.
- Once something is online, it can be copied and redistributed.
- If unsure whether something you have posted online could compromise your professionalism or your reputation, think

about what the information means for you in practice and how it affects your responsibility to adhere to the Code.
- It is important to consider who and what you associate with on social media; for example, acknowledging someone else's post could suggest that you endorse or support their point of view.
- Consider the possibility of other people mentioning you in inappropriate posts.
- Think, in relation to the Code, what you have posted online in the past.

Source: Adapted NMC (2019).

If you have any concerns about your fitness to practise or your ability to aspire to the tenets within the Code and other guidance, you should seek support and help from your practice assessor, academic assessor (university tutor) or practice supervisor straight away. They can provide you with the support and advice that you may need before the matter becomes a more serious issue. Support services may include confidential counselling, disability advisers, supervisors, occupational health services, personal tutors, professional bodies or trade unions, student groups or unions, or student health services.

Over to you

Ask for help if needed.

To make sure that you are always able to access all the help and advice you need, be sure to familiarise yourself with the student support services available within your university and those located within the clinical placement.

Professional regulation and the professional register

Professional regulation is intended to protect the public, making sure that those who practise a health or care profession are doing so safely. Employers have a duty to check the registration of healthcare professionals with the relevant regulatory body. It is usually a contractual condition of employment that the health or care professional has registration throughout their term of employment. The NMC can provide registration information on registered nurses and midwives and will inform an employer if a practitioner has the following status:

- removed
- restored
- conditions of practice
- cautioned
- suspended
- lapsed
- effective.

The NMC register shows who can practise as a nurse or midwife in the UK, or in England as a nursing associate. Anyone can search the NMC register. The details of registrants include those who:

- Have effective registration with no restrictions and cautions, with registration fees having been paid and registration is up to date.
- Are on the register but have restrictions on their practice or a caution order.
- Have been suspended or removed from the register since 1 January 2008 and are not currently permitted to practice.

The parts of the register

The legislation governing the NMC is set out in the Nursing and Midwifery Order 2001. It requires that the NMC establishes and maintains a register and determines the standards of proficiency that are required to be admitted to the different parts of that register. The NMC register is divided into parts, each of which has a title indicative of the qualifications, education or training necessary to be on that part. When a name is entered on the register, this permits the nurse, midwife or nursing associate to use the title corresponding to the part in which they are registered.

Red flag

It an offence for someone to falsely represent themselves as being on the register, or on a part of it, to use a title to which they are not entitled or to falsely represent themselves as having qualifications in nursing or midwifery.

These provisions, when taken together, make it a legal requirement for any nurse or midwife who is practising in the UK or any nursing associate practising in England to be on the NMC register. There are three broad parts to the register:

1. Nurses part of the register subpart 1:
   - Adult nurse, level 1
   - Mental health nurse, level 1
   - Learning disabilities nurse, level 1
   - Children's nurse, level 1
2. Nurses part of the register subpart 2:
   - Adult nurse, level 2
   - Mental health nurse, level 2
   - Learning disabilities nurse, level 2
   - General nurse, level 2
   - Fever nurse, level 2
3. Nursing associates part of the register:
   - Nursing associate
4. Midwives part of the register:
   - Midwife
5. Specialist community public health nursing part of the register:
   - Health visitor
   - School nurse
   - Occupational health nurse
   - Family health nurse
   - Specialist community public health nurse.

There is also a range of qualifications that are known as recordable qualifications.

How to search the register

Searching the register is free. All those on the register are given a unique registration code: their personal identification number or PIN. A nurse, midwife or nursing associate is required to provide details of their PIN by a person who is using their services when asked. If, when searching the register, the PIN is not known the search can be made by using the first and last name, this could however, return more than one result.

The following details are shown for the person being searched for:

- name
- registration status
- geographical location
- expiry date

- register entry
- start date
- recorded qualifications.

Different terms are used by the NMC to describe the registration status of those on the register (Table 1.1).

TABLE 1.1

Glossary of terms used to describe a person's registration status.

Term	Meaning
Registered	The nurse, midwife or nursing associate is on the register with no restrictions or cautions.
Not currently practising	The nurse, midwife, or nursing associate has informed the NMC that they are no longer practising, however, they remain on the register until their current registration period expires.
Removed by a fitness to practise (FtP) panel	The nurse, midwife or nursing associate is not permitted to practise if they have been struck off or removed from the register.
Suspended by an FtP panel	The nurse, midwife or nursing associate is not permitted to practise if they have been suspended from the register for a fixed period. The suspension order will be reviewed prior to it expiring and it may be replaced or revoked.
Voluntarily removed	The nurse, midwife or nursing associate is not permitted to practise if they have admitted that their fitness to practise is impaired and they have no intention of practising again. They can request to have their name voluntarily removed from the register.
Interim suspension order	The nurse, midwife or nursing associate is not permitted to practise, following the making of an interim suspension order by an FtP panel. This remains in place while the NMC is investigating allegations about the person's fitness to practise or pending an appeal. This interim suspension order will be regularly reviewed and may be replaced or revoked.
Conditions of practice order	The circumstances under which the nurse, midwife or nursing associate on the register can practise are restricted following a final order by an FtP panel. These conditions may be in place for one to three years. They are reviewed before they expire and may be replaced, varied or revoked.

TABLE 1.1	

(Continued)

Term	Meaning
Interim conditions	The circumstances under which someone on the register can practise are currently restricted following the making of an interim conditions of practice order. This will remain while the NMC investigate allegations about the person's fitness to practise or pending an appeal. These conditions will be regularly reviewed and may be replaced, varied or revoked.
Undertakings	Undertakings are agreed measures to address areas of practice which cause a current clinical risk to patients. Undertakings include steps that should be taken within defined time periods to demonstrate remediation. If undertakings are agreed, they will be published on the register in all cases, together with a brief summary of the regulatory concern (except in cases relating to health).
Sanction pending	This is where a nurse, midwife or nursing associate has had a final sanction imposed on them by a fitness to practise panel but it will not take effect until the end of a 28-day appeal period or the outcome of any appeal. The person's practice may be restricted by an interim order in the meantime.
Caution order	A caution order is where someone on the register is permitted to practise without any restriction but has been made the subject of a caution order following a final order by an FtP panel. This can last from between one and five years.
Warnings	This is a public marking (on the register) of serious concerns about someone on the register without the need for a hearing. Warnings are only appropriate where the individual shows insight, remediation, and there is no risk to patients. Warnings will be published for 12 months on the register, including a short summary of the regulatory concern.
No recorded qualifications found	This means an individual has no additional qualifications added to their registration, for example, lecturer/practice educator, teacher, V200, nurse independent prescriber

Source: Adapted from NMC (2020).

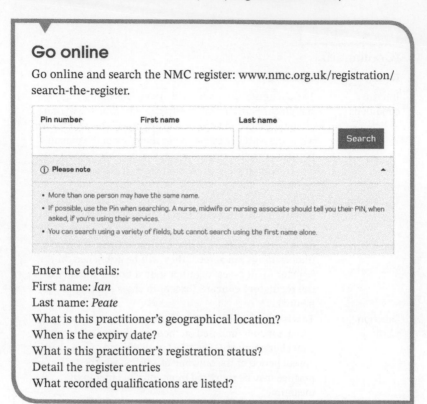

Go online

Go online and search the NMC register: www.nmc.org.uk/registration/ search-the-register.

Pin number	First name	Last name	
			Search

ⓘ **Please note** ▲

- More than one person may have the same name.
- If possible, use the Pin when searching. A nurse, midwife or nursing associate should tell you their PIN, when asked, if you're using their services.
- You can search using a variety of fields, but cannot search using the first name alone.

Enter the details:
First name: *Ian*
Last name: *Peate*
What is this practitioner's geographical location?
When is the expiry date?
What is this practitioner's registration status?
Detail the register entries
What recorded qualifications are listed?

Programme validation and approval

It has been discussed previously that your name will only be entered onto the professional register when you have successfully completed all parts of the NMC approved programme and met all of the conditions required. There are a number of complex and robust procedures that approved institutions must complete prior to the NMC approving a programme that leads to registration.

A series of ambitious standards were published by the NMC in May 2018, as part of the regulator's new standards for education and future nurse plans (Chapter 2 of this text provides more detail of these standards). The introduction of these standards has resulted in significant changes to the education and preparation of those undertaking NMC approved programmes of study.

While the standards impact on students and those who provide education (practice partners and universities), they will also have implications for the people who nurses care for and will affect the whole of the nursing workforce. The changing demographics (locally, nationally and internationally) and developments in healthcare priorities prompted a change and the standards of proficiency needed to be ambitious to meet the needs of populations now and in the future; they needed to be future proofed. The standards are the blueprint for how universities devise and develop curricula.

Try this on placement

When you are in placement, take some time to consider, within that area of care, what are the key demographic changes. For example, has this care area seen an increase in older people accessing this service? Has there been an increase in people generally accessing the service?

The programme you are currently undertaking would not have been able to run until it had successfully passed through the NMCs approval processes and the NMC had confirmed in writing that it had been approved. The educational institution offering the programme would also have had to have gone through a number of internal processes of its own so as to ensure that it meets all of the university's specifications.

The NMC will make an approval based on whether education institutions, as well as their practice learning partners, can meet the education and training standards and also the relevant programme standards. Approval comes after a four-part process has been undertaken and the education institution has demonstrated that it has met the NMC's demanding standards. Once approved the institution becomes known as an approved education institution (AEI).

An AEI is the status that is awarded to an institution, part of an institution or combination of institutions working in partnership with practice placements and work placed learning providers. AEIs are required to have provided the NMC with assurance that they are accountable and able to deliver NMC approved education programmes.

Go online

Using the dropdown menu, go online and search for an approved nursing or nursing associate education programme: www.nmc.org.uk/education/approved-programmes.

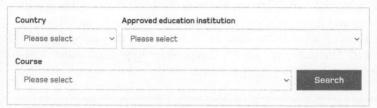

This search facility shows programmes that offer a formal qualification from the NMC's approved education providers.

While the NMC sets the standards that AEIs must keep, as well as the standards that student nurses must meet to enter and stay on the register, it does not set the curriculum that students follow; individual AEIs are responsible for designing and developing these curricula. The NMCs pre-registration nursing standards include:

- The minimum length of nursing pre-registration programmes.
- The criteria to be met at various progression points.
- The core proficiencies that all students must meet for them to progress through their programme and gain entry into the register.

The pre-registration nursing standards include specific guidance that are related to each of the four pre-registration nursing specialisms:

- adult
- children
- learning disabilities
- mental health.

As well as the standards relating to the four nursing specialisms (fields; field specific), all pre-registration nursing programmes include standards for students to care for all patient groups (generic). All registered nurses are expected to be able to deal with the majority of nursing roles regardless of field.

Quality assurance

There are several quality assurance processes that the NMC has in place to ensure that those who are offering or wish to offer nurse education programmes are doing this according to legal and governance principles. Public safety is at the core of the NMC's standards. As students will be in contact with people throughout the duration of their educational programme, it is therefore essential that any learning must be carried out in a safe, supportive and effective way.

The quality of the learning experience to which students are exposed is the responsibility of the AEIs, as they are working in partnership with practice learning partners, managing the quality of the educational programme. Important issues such as these are clear in the various NMC educational standards.

Standards framework for nursing and midwifery education

These standards (NMC 2019) are set against a framework that allows the flexibility to develop creative and innovative approaches to education that will be responsive to local and national needs, as well as ensuring that institutions remain accountable for the local delivery and management of approved programmes Table 1.2 gives an overview of the standards framework.

Processes are implemented by the NMC as it checks that education programmes meet the standards and that education institutions and practice learning partners are managing any risks effectively. Data are collected, analysed and responded to with regards to risk, including any concerns that are raised directly with the NMC by students. Education providers must self-report any risks or concerns that have the potential to affect the quality of programme delivery and as such, public protection.

TABLE 1.2

The standards framework.

Component	Discussion
Learning culture	Approval is only made where the learning culture is ethical, open and honest, and lends itself to safe and effective learning, respecting the principles of equality and diversity. Innovation, interprofessional learning and teamworking should be embedded in the learning culture.
Education governance and quality	Education providers must comply with all legal and regulatory requirements. These include, for example, legislation regarding health and safety at work, the Equality Act and data protection legislation.
Student empowerment	The AEI must be able to demonstrate that they can provide learning opportunities so that students can achieve the desired proficiencies and programme outcomes.
Educators and assessors	Ensuring that that those who support, supervise, and assess students are suitably qualified, are appropriately prepared and skilled and receive the necessary support so that they can undertake their role.
Curricula and assessment	Curricula and assessment have to be provided in such a way that it enables students to achieve the outcomes needed so they will be able to practise safely and effectively in their chosen area.

Source: Adapted NMC (2018b).

Complete this activity now

Write notes/provide definitions of the following terms.

Term	Notes/definition
Approved education institution	
Educators	
Learning environment	
Practice learning partner	
Service user	
Student	

These standards (Table 1.2) should be read in conjunction with:

- Part 2: Standards for Student Supervision and Assessment (NMC 2018c). These standards set out the NMC's expectations for the learning, support and supervision of students in the practice environment. They also set out how students are assessed for theory and practice learning.
- Part 3: Programme standards:
  - Standards for Pre-registration Nursing Education (NMC 2018d)
  - Standards for Pre-registration Nursing Associates (NMC 2018e)

Together, these are the NMC Standards for Education and Training for Nursing.

The standards of proficiency

The standards of proficiency for registered nurses (NMC 2018f) and the standards of proficiency for registered nursing associates (NMC 2018g) set out the knowledge and skills that registered nurses and registered nursing associates must meet. The standards are arranged under platforms and annexes. Chapter 2 of this text considers the standards of proficiency in more detail.

University programme approval

As discussed, the NMC has its own processes and procedures in place to ensure that the nurse whose name is to be entered on the register has met all of its stringent requirements. The student who is to receive an academic award (e.g. a degree) must also demonstrate to the awarding body that they have met the standards that will merit the academic award.

Programme design and development is a complex activity. Programme (or curriculum) designers also have to ensure that any professional, regulatory and statutory body standards are incorporated into the programme. Curricula and assessment feature in the NMC's Standards Framework (NMC 2018b).

Programmes that terminate in an academic award must be well-designed, provide a high-quality academic experience for all students

Hear it from the student

Hello my name is Jacques; I was a second-year learning disability student when my tutor at the uni asked me to join a curriculum planning group. There were four students all together, from all four fields. We are now at the end of our third year, close to registration.

When I joined this group, it really opened my eyes into the work, effort and attention to detail that is required to have a programme approved by not only the NMC but also by the uni itself. The head of school informed us that the student contribution is invaluable for future educational improvement and ultimately the patient experience. There was so much reading to do but I learned so much about regulation, the regulatory process and the role and function of the NMC, I know now where my registration fee will be going!

I would say if anyone asks you, or even if you asked to be included, to join a planning group – then go for it. You will come away with deeper insight as to what goes on behind the scenes. I am about to qualify and I am now seeing first-year students on the programme that I helped to develop – a nice feeling.

Jacques, third year learning disability nursing field

and enable a student's achievement to be reliably assessed. Standards are set and monitored by organisations such as the Quality Assurance Agency (QAA 2019).

Write here

What is the role and function of the Quality Assurance Agency?

Registration with the Nursing and Midwifery Council

While it may seem like a long way off for some, when the time comes for registration with the NMC, there are a number of things that you need to do before your name is entered on the register. The responsibility will be on you to address these issues.

For those who have successfully completed an approved programme of study that leads to registration in the UK, the AEI will upload your programme and personal details to the NMC database. The AEI is also required to send a declaration of your good health and character. When everything from the AEI has been received, a letter will be sent to you telling you how to create your online NMC account.

Once you have applied online and paid your registration fee, your application is then reviewed. You must declare any police cautions or criminal convictions (Box 1.2). If everything is in order, your name will be entered onto the register within 2–10 working days.

If you make your application for entry into the register more than six months after finishing your programme, the NMC will require further

Box 1.2 | Police cautions or criminal convictions

Universities are required to have regulations and a detailed process for the consideration of applications for courses leading to professional registration that require enhanced disclosure. For those students on courses that lead to professional registration, universities must consider all convictions as these are exempt from the provisions of the Rehabilitation of Offenders Act (1974). The declaration of a criminal offence (including convictions, cautions, reprimands or warnings) is not in itself a bar to entry on the programme. However, any offence will be considered together with the applicant's qualifications, experience and overall profile, as well as any professional or statutory body requirements.

If, as a student, you receive a caution or conviction, you should inform the appropriate person at your university prior to it being revealed in a future disclosure and barring service certificate. The programme provider (the AEI) must consider how the caution or conviction may impact on your nursing. The AEI is acting on behalf of the NMC when it selects students and must always make decisions with public protection in mind.

When you apply to register for the first time, you will also need to personally inform the NMC about any convictions, cautions or matters relating to your character. You cannot rely on the university to do this for you.

information. You will need to provide a further reference from a registered nurse. If you apply more than five years after finishing your programme, different standards will apply and you are required to contact the NMC.

Summary

This chapter has introduced the reader to the issues that are associated with programme construction and content. It is of value to understand the intricacies and the complexities that are related to the design and development of your programme. This may go some way to explaining why there are some specific requirements of your programme that have to be met that are an absolute requirement. Having insight can assist you as you make your journey through the convolutions of nurse education.

The NMC, whose key role is to protect the public and is required by law to set the standards for programmes that lead to entry into the professional register, has dominated discussion in this chapter. The various standards have been discussed, highlighting the robust and stringent measures that AEIs must demonstrate to receive NMC approval.

The regulatory process has been discussed in detail and the important issue of maintaining a professional register. The NMC is robust in the way they maintain and manage the register and have statutory obligations that they must enact when a nurse fails to meet the standards required, these standards are detailed in the Code.

References

General Medical Council (2014). Openness and Honesty – the Professional Duty of Candour: Joint Statement from the Chief Executives of Statutory Regulators of Healthcare Professionals. www.pharmacyregulation.org/sites/default/files/joint_statement_on_the_professional_duty_of_candour.pdf (accessed March 2023).

McGrath, L., Swift, A., Clark, M. et al. (2019). Understanding the benefits and risks of nursing students engaging with online social media. *Nursing Standard* 34 (10): 45–49. https://doi.org/10.7748/ns.2019.e11362.

Nursing and Midwifery Council (2018a). The Code: Professional Standards of Practice and Behaviour for Nurses, Midwives and Nursing Associates. www.nmc.org.uk/standards/code (accessed December 2020).

Nursing and Midwifery Council (2018b). Realising Professionalism: Standards for Education and Training. Part 1: Standards Framework for Nursing and Midwifery Education.

www.nmc.org.uk/globalassets/sitedocuments/education-standards/education-framework.pdf (accessed December 2020).

Nursing and Midwifery Council (2018c). Realising Professionalism: Standards for Education and Training. Part 2: Standards for Student Supervision and Assessment. www.nmc.org.uk/Student-supervision-assessment (accessed December 2020).

Nursing and Midwifery Council (2018d). Realising Professionalism: Standards for Education and Training. Part 3: Standards for Pre-registration Nursing Education. www.nmc.org.uk/Programme-standards-nursing (accessed December 2020).

Nursing and Midwifery Council (2018e). Realising Professionalism: Standards for Education and Training: Standards for Pre-registration Nursing Associate Programmes. www.nmc.org.uk/programme-standards-nursing (accessed December 2020).

Nursing and Midwifery Council (2018f). Future Nurse: The Standards of Proficiency for Registered Nurses. www.nmc.org.uk/globalassets/sitedocuments/education-standards/future-nurse-proficiencies.pdf (accessed December 2020).

Nursing and Midwifery Council (2018g). Standards of Proficiency for Registered Nursing Associates. www.nmc.org.uk/standards/standards-for-nursing-associates/standards-of-proficiency-for-nursing-associates (accessed December 2020).

Nursing and Midwifery Council (2019). Guidance on Using Social Media Responsibly. https://www.nmc.org.uk/globalassets/sitedocuments/nmc-publications/social-media-guidance.pdf (accessed December 2020).

Nursing and Midwifery Council (2020). How to Search the Register: A Glossary of Terms used in the Search the Register Results. www.nmc.org.uk/registration/search-the-register/how-to-use-search-the-register (accessed December 2020).

Nursing and Midwifery Council (2022a). The NMC Register England Mid-year Update 1 April – 30 September 2022. www.nmc.org.uk/globalassets/sitedocuments/data-reports/sep-2022/0082e-mid-year-report-england-web.pdf (accessed March 2023).

Nursing and Midwifery Council (2022b). The NMC Register Scotland Mid-year Update 1 April – 30 September 2022. www.nmc.org.uk/globalassets/sitedocuments/data-reports/sep-2022/0082d-mid-year-report-scotland-web.pdf (accessed March 2023).

Nursing and Midwifery Council (2022c). The NMC Register Wales Mid-year Update 1 April – 30 September 2022. www.nmc.org.uk/globalassets/sitedocuments/data-reports/sep-2022/0082c-mid-year-report-wales-web.pdf (accessed March 2023).

Quality Assurance Agency (2019). UK Quality Code for Higher Education: Advice and Guidance: Course Design and Development. www.qaa.ac.uk/the-quality-code/advice-and-guidance/course-design-and-development (accessed December 2020).

CHAPTER 2

The Nursing and Midwifery Council standards

Scott Rodden and Ian Peate

AIM

This chapter presents an overview of the Nursing and Midwifery Council (NMC) standards of proficiency.

LEARNING OUTCOMES

Having read this chapter, the reader will:

1. Be able to demonstrate an awareness of the NMC's standards of proficiency.
2. Understand how a programme of study is constructed using the standards of proficiency as a framework.
3. Be aware of the various requirements that are detailed in the standards of proficiency.
4. Be able to describe how the standards will impact a student's progression throughout their nursing programme.

Succeeding on your Nursing Placement: Supervision, Learning and Assessment for Nursing Students, First Edition. Edited by Ian Peate.
© 2024 John Wiley & Sons Ltd. Published 2024 by John Wiley & Sons Ltd.

Introduction

In Chapter 1, the role and function of the NMC is detailed. As discussed, the NMC is required to provide details of programme requirements that will enable a student, at the end of successfully completing all components of their programme, to have their name entered into the professional register. The standards of proficiency represent the standards of knowledge and skills that a registered nurse or a nursing associate is required to meet so that the NMC can determine if they are considered safe and effective in the delivery of nursing care.

This chapter outlines the various NMC standards with a focus on the standards of proficiency for registered nurses and nursing associates (NMC 2018a,b). The contents of these seminal documents are discussed (Figure 2.1).

A supervisor's notes

I went on a study day/update informing our community nursing team of the various standards that the NMC has put together. The changes are important; there was a need to introduce change to ensure that the next generation of nurses can deal with the demands of the role, as well as what we want the profession to look like as we move forward. A big part of this change required universities who train nurses to change and make sure that the nurses of tomorrow have the skills they need to provide safe and high-quality care. The introduction of the NMC standards impact all of us and, most importantly, the patient and their family.

The standards

After a two-year process and working alongside key stakeholders including students, educators, health professionals, independent sector organisations, charities and patient groups from across the UK, the NMC introduced a suite of new standards. The standards consist of three parts (Table 2.1).

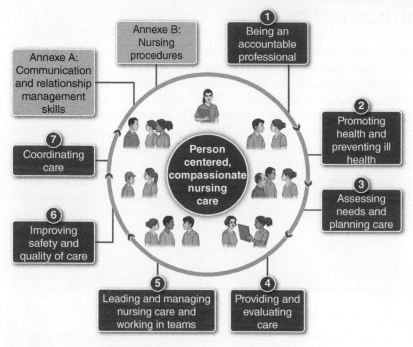

FIGURE 2.1 Future nurse proficiencies.

TABLE 2.1

The NMC.

Part	Content
1	Standards framework for nursing and midwifery education containing five sections underpinning nurse education and training: 1. Learning culture 2. Educational governance and quality 3. Student learning and empowerment 4. Educators and assessors 5. Curricula and assessment
2	These are the standards for student supervision and assessment, setting out the expectations for learning, support, supervision and assessment (of theory and practice) of students in the practice environment
3	The programme standards are specific to each pre-registration or post-registration programme. Here, the legislative requirements for all pre-registration nursing education programmes can be found.

The nursing workforce

Nurses are central to the effective delivery of health and social care services. They work across hospitals, community services, care homes and within the primary care setting. The NHS employs the majority of nurses in hospital and community services, and it is nurses who make up approximately one quarter of all NHS staff (National Audit Office 2020).

While the majority of nurses and health care support workers working in the independent sector are located in nursing and care homes, the sector covers a wide range of workplaces including hospices, general practice surgeries, private hospitals, charities and voluntary community services. The businesses include privately owned companies, charitable institutions and social enterprises. Private sector independent healthcare organisations provide a significant amount of long-term care within the UK, often to help reduce the strain on the NHS, as well as reducing waiting times. Most private-sector care is run by profit organisations. Other employment opportunities could include schools and universities, or organisations that require in-house medical professionals (e.g. the services of an occupational health nurse).

Hear it from the student

As part of our uni induction we met with second and third year students via Zoom so we could share and support each other. Each of the current students shared with us how the programme was going; they all said it was tough and not all a bed of roses. By far the best part of it, they all agreed, was the clinical placements. What really surprised me was the range of placements that are available and the places where nurses are working. One of the students has been doing mental health outreach work with the homeless during the COVID pandemic – amazing. I just wonder, will I be able to meet the challenges that they have faced?

Amble, first-year mental health field student nurse

It has been acknowledged throughout the UK that there is a need to increase staff numbers across the NHS. The biggest shortfalls being seen in nursing (NHS England 2019) were recognised in 2017; the NHS does not have the nurses it needs. The majority of nurses work in acute, elderly and general settings. Others work in community services, community mental health, other mental health settings, paediatric settings, neonatal and learning disabilities. It must be remembered that sometimes nurses work in more than one setting; for example, a nurse may work in a neonatal unit and a paediatric care setting.

The major source of nurses entering the NMC register do so via the graduate route. Undergraduate courses are usually three years in duration, with half the time spent in the classroom (at least 2300 hours) and half the time (at least 2300 hours) on clinical placement. Student nurses on clinical placement work in a number of health and care settings under supervision, to gain practical experience and apply theory to practice.

Try this on placement

When you are in a clinical area (or even when you are at the university) find out if there are any nursing associates and apprenticeship nurses working with you. If you identify anyone, chat with them about their experiences on the programme, compare and contrast your own situation with theirs.

Apprenticeships and nursing associates

A new apprenticeship-based route into nursing has been developed. Nursing degree apprenticeships have been available since 2017. In contrast to those students on nursing degrees, healthcare providers employ nursing degree apprentices while they work and train, including external study at an approved education institution. Apprentices study for four years towards a nursing degree.

A new nursing associate role was introduced in January 2017, aimed at bridging the gap between registered nurses and healthcare assistants. Intended as a role in its own right that can free up registered nurses to carry out more advanced roles, another objective was to develop a new route into nursing. Nursing associate training is two years and leads to a level 5 qualification (e.g. a foundation degree). To become a registered nurse, a nursing associate must study for around a further two years to 'top up' their qualification.

Apprenticeships and nursing associate roles are potentially a more accessible, if longer, route to becoming a registered nurse (House of

Commons 2020). Apprenticeships and nursing associates play an important role in widening access to the nursing profession. This route enables you to earn money as you train. Nursing associates can gain experience as an associate prior to deciding if they want to train to become a registered nurse.

As you embark on your nursing course you will meet student nurses who have taken a different route to gaining their NMC registration. Student nurses have two routes available to them when considering their nurse education:

- Route 1: attending university as a full-time nursing student.
- Route 2: attending university part time as an apprentice.

Nursing apprentices are employed by an NHS trust or another healthcare provider, such as a nursing home or a doctor's surgery. Apprentices can study to be a registered nurse or a registered nursing associate. As nursing apprentices are employed and sponsored to undertake their studies, they are required to work alongside their study. There are some fundamental differences between a nursing student who studies full time and a nursing apprentice, a full time nursing student and a nursing apprentice (Table 2.2).

Nursing apprenticeships in the UK are only delivered by accredited education institutions that are approved by the NMC. Additionally, those studying on an apprenticeship course may come across Ofsted inspectors during your programme, as Ofsted inspects apprenticeship programmes to ensure that they meet government apprenticeship standards (Department for Education 2022). As the landscape of pre-registration nurse education continues to grow, the types of education institutions delivering nursing courses is changing. Traditionally, nursing degrees were run by public universities, whereas now there are private universities providing nurse education programmes. Public universities are beginning to work with local further education institutions, creating local partnerships allowing nursing degrees and apprenticeships that will benefit the local community.

Whichever route chosen or the type of educational institution you choose for your studies, the outcome remains the same upon successful completion: entry to the NMC register within your field of nursing.

The proficiencies

Within the dynamic and complex environment of health and care provision, the nurse's experience and expertise are contributing factors to the quality of care and positive patient outcomes. The concept of clinical

---

TABLE **2.2**

A full time nursing student and a nursing apprentice.

Full time student nurse	Nursing apprentice
Attends university on a full-time basis	Attends university part time and is required to work a contracted number of hours in their normal role
Has holidays built into their timetable	Entitled to annual leave with allocated times within the timetable were this can be booked
Will have one to one sessions or tutorials with their named tutor	Will have one to one sessions or tutorials with their named tutor; the apprentice's manager may be involved in this process
Three-year programme	Four-year programme for registered nurse apprentice; two-year programme for registered nurse associates
Interviewed for entry to the programme by the university	Interviewed for entry to the programme by the employer and the university
Will complete assessments in theory and practice placements	Will complete theory assessments and practice placements, and will undertake an endpoint assessment at the end of the programme to ensure that all programme requirement have been met, which will be a pass or fail (Education and Skills Funding Agency 2022)

---

nursing expertise is closely related to proficiency and is central to quality patient care. It follows therefore that the student must be assessed against set criteria that makes a judgement concerning their performance. To be successful in a nursing programme, the student has to demonstrate proficiency when being assessed in the practice setting, which is usually a pass or fail grade. The theoretical component of the programme is also assessed, with the student receiving a percentage grade mark that is set against specific criteria.

The assessment of the nursing student's clinical competence is complex and can bring with it challenges. There are a number of factors that impact on the student clinical assessment, including the clinical learning environment and the quality of the supervision provided, as well as the support structures that are in place to help guide the learning. It can, however, be difficult to define competence and difficult to measure it reliably. Immonen et al. (2019) call for consistent and systematic approaches to assessing competence in practice.

Complete this activity now

Provide a definition for these two terms (related to the performance of a clinical skill):

• Competence

• Proficiency

The provision of clear assessment criteria is key to helping those who undertake the assessment of clinical performance, as it is for the student who is being subjected to the assessment. Consistent and systematic approaches to assessment are required, together with the use of reliable and valid instruments. Observation of student performance and the use of skills checklists are common approaches to assessment and observations of structured clinical examination (OSCE). The various types of assessment can be formative or summative.

Write here

Within your programme make a list of the assignments that you have that are:

Formative	Summative

Formative assessment is a continuing process; it lasts throughout clinical education and is based on feedback given by others (e.g. supervisors and assessors). Its purpose is to assist the student towards a goal. Formative assessment aims to prepare students for the summative assessment; this assessment is usually undertaken at the end of the module.

Standards of proficiency for registered nurses and registered nursing associates

These standards indicate the knowledge and skills expected from nursing professionals when caring for people across the lifespan in various care settings with consideration to ethnicity and social status. The role of registered nurses requires them to be people centred, compassionate, and with a desire to offer care and support to people eager to render care for those who depend on them.

Registered nurses have an essential role to play in providing care and promoting safety, making a contribution to the promotion of quality health for all. Nurses are seen at the forefront of health protection and the prevention of ill health empowering people, communities and populations to take control of their own health decisions for healthy living.

Nurses are required to provide evidence-based, compassionate care interventions that are consistent with the standards of proficiency. They also evaluate whether the care provided to people is aligned to their needs and preferences, and has been effective. Table 2.3 shows a snapshot of the seven platforms within the standards of proficiency for registered nurses.

The nursing associate proficiencies are similar to those for the registered nurse. There are six platforms for these practitioners:

1. Being an accountable professional.
2. Promoting health and preventing ill health.
3. Providing and monitoring care.
4. Working in teams.
5. Improving safety and quality of care.
6. Contributing to integrated care.

Over to you

Take some time out and look at the six platforms that are related to the nursing associate proficiencies and the seven platforms related to the registered nurse. Think about what makes them different and why.

People who use health and care services will benefit from the care that is given by nursing associates in a range of settings. While the NMC does not set out what a nursing associate can and cannot do (this is the role of the employer), it does ensure that they are able to demonstrate the knowledge and skills required as defined in the standards (NMC 2018b) to deliver better, safer care prior to entering the workforce. The nursing associate (just like their registered nurse counterpart) can enhance their knowledge and skills aligned to their scope of practice throughout their professional career.

> **TABLE 2.3**

Standards of proficiency for registered nurses.

Platform	Overview
Being an accountable professional	The role of registered nurses implies that they are accountable for their actions and must always act in the best interests of those they offer care and support to. Being accountable also means that the nurse will act professionally at all times, making use of their knowledge and experience as they make correct evidence-based choices regarding care. They are expected to be people centred, providing safe and compassionate nursing care at every given time. The registered nurse must also have high-quality communication skills, effectively communicating with patients and colleagues. They must act as role models for others and be responsible for their actions at all times, with the aim of constant improvements in their sphere of practice and beyond.
Promoting health and preventing ill health	Registered nurses are key players in improving and maintaining health. They have essential roles to play in helping others to maintain quality mental, physical and behavioural health, and to promote healthy living and preventing ill health among communities and populations at all stages of life and in all care settings. Registered nurses are at the forefront of preventing and controlling diseases.
Assessing needs, planning care	Registered nurses assess and prioritise the needs of people when reviewing their health. Nurses, working with patients (and, if appropriate, with others) assess patients to identify what needs people may have from a variety of perspectives, including mental, physical, cognitive, behavioural, social or spiritual.
Providing and evaluating care	When assessment has been undertaken, the nurse works hand in hand with the patients and other healthcare professionals to develop person-centred care plans according to the needs of the patients. Evaluation of interventions is a key component of the nurse's role.
Leading and managing nursing care and working in teams	Registered nurses provide leadership by acting as role models for best practice in the delivery of nursing care. They are responsible for managing nursing care and are accountable for the appropriate delegation and supervision of care provided by others in the team, including lay carers. They play an active and equal role in the interdisciplinary team, collaborating and communicating effectively with a range of colleagues.

(Continued)

TABLE **2.3**

(Continued)

Platform	Overview
Improving safety and quality of care	Registered nurses make a key contribution to the continuous monitoring and quality improvement of care and treatment to enhance health outcomes and people's experience of nursing and related care. They assess risks to safety or experience and take appropriate action to manage those, putting the best interests, needs and preferences of people first.
Coordinating care	Registered nurses play a leadership role in coordinating and managing the complex nursing and integrated care needs of people at any stage of their lives, across a range of organisations and settings. They contribute to processes of organisational change through an awareness of local and national policies.

Source: Adapted from NMC (2018a).

Green flag

It should be noted that a nursing associate is not permitted to prescribe.

While the nursing associate contributes to most aspects of care, including delivery and monitoring, it is the registered nurse who takes the lead with regards to assessment, planning and evaluation. Registered nurses will take the lead on managing and coordinating care with full support from the nursing associate, working together as a part of an integrated care team.

Go online

Access the standards for the nursing associate and the registered nurse at:

www.nmc.org.uk/standards/standards-for-nursing-associates/standards-of-proficiency-for-nursing-associates

and for the registered nurse at:

www.nmc.org.uk/globalassets/sitedocuments/education-standards/future-nurse-proficiencies.pdf

Bookmark these pages, as you may need to access them at a later date.

The platforms

The six platforms within the standards of proficiency for registered nurses (NMC 2018a) are detailed here. Understanding what these platforms contain and what is expected of the student, can help to provide insight into practice-based requirements for your programme of study.

> ### Green flag
>
> The proficiencies define precisely what the student's training will require them to know and what it is that they are permitted to do.

The outcome statements associated with each of the platforms have been constructed in such a way that they apply across all health and care. Registered nurses must be able to meet the person-centred holistic care needs of those people with whom they come into contact in their practice. These people may be at any stage of life and who may also have a range of mental, physical, cognitive or behavioural health challenges.

To reiterate at the point of registration, the student must meet all of the outcome statements and also demonstrate an awareness of them ensuring that they are safe and proficient. Box 2.1, shows the full outcome statement for Platform 1 (NMC 2018a); there are 20 outcome statements in total.

> ### How to
>
> Outcome statement 1.4 requires you to demonstrate an understanding of, and the ability to challenge, discriminatory behaviour. Promoting equality and respecting diversity are central to the role and function of the nurse; they are not only professional requirements, they are also legal requirements. When you are offering care and support to people, you must ensure that it meets the needs of everyone. Equality and respecting diversity must be taken into account in all aspects of your work.
>
> Equality focuses on treating people alike, responsive to their needs. Everyone should be given equality of opportunity. It could be that there

is a requirement to provide information in different formats (e.g. large print or a need to ensure that those who use wheelchairs are able to access buildings and use equipment). Diversity is concerned with 'difference'. All of us are different; the different parts of a person's character and identity (and there are many of these) make them unique. Some of the things that make people different are:

- health status
- background
- gender
- family
- friends
- sexual orientation
- religion
- belief
- values

- culture
- race
- national origins
- marital status
- age
- appearance
- ability
- disability
- job role

Box 2.1 | The 20 outcome statements associated with platform one of the standards

At the point of registration, the registered nurse will be able to:

1.1 understand and act in accordance with the Code: professional standards of practice and behaviour for nurses, midwives and nursing associates, and fulfil all registration requirements.

1.2 understand and apply relevant legal, regulatory and governance requirements, policies, and ethical frameworks, including any mandatory reporting duties, to all areas of practice, differentiating where appropriate between the devolved legislatures of the United Kingdom.

1.3 understand and apply the principles of courage, transparency and the professional duty of candour, recognising and reporting any situations, behaviours or errors that could result in poor care outcomes.

1.4 demonstrate an understanding of, and the ability to challenge, discriminatory behaviour.

1.5 understand the demands of professional practice and demonstrate how to recognise signs of vulnerability in themselves or their colleagues and the action required to minimise risks to health.

1.6 understand the professional responsibility to adopt a healthy lifestyle to maintain the level of personal fitness and wellbeing required to meet people's needs for mental and physical care.

1.7 demonstrate an understanding of research methods, ethics and governance in order to critically analyse, safely use, share and apply research findings to promote and inform best nursing practice.

1.8 demonstrate the knowledge, skills and ability to think critically when applying evidence and drawing on experience to make evidence informed decisions in all situations.

1.9 understand the need to base all decisions regarding care and interventions on people's needs and preferences, recognising and addressing any personal and external factors that may unduly influence their decisions.

1.10 demonstrate resilience and emotional intelligence and be capable of explaining the rationale that influences their judgements and decisions in routine, complex and challenging situations.

1.11 communicate effectively using a range of skills and strategies with colleagues and people at all stages of life and with a range of mental, physical, cognitive and behavioural health.

1.12 demonstrate the skills and abilities required to support people at all stages of life who are emotionally or physically vulnerable.

1.13 demonstrate the skills and abilities required to develop, manage and maintain appropriate relationships with people, their families, carers and colleagues.

1.14 provide and promote non-discriminatory, person centred and sensitive care at all times, reflecting on people's values and beliefs, diverse backgrounds, cultural characteristics, language requirements, needs and preferences, taking account of any need for adjustments.

1.15 demonstrate the numeracy, literacy, digital and technological skills required to meet the needs of people in their care to ensure safe and effective nursing practice.

1.16 demonstrate the ability to keep complete, clear, accurate and timely records.

1.17 take responsibility for continuous self-reflection, seeking and responding to support and feedback to develop their professional knowledge and skills.

1.18 demonstrate the knowledge and confidence to contribute effectively and proactively in an interdisciplinary team.

1.19 act as an ambassador, upholding the reputation of their profession and promoting public confidence in nursing, health and care services.

1.20 safely demonstrate evidence-based practice in all skills and procedures stated in Annexes A and B.

Source: Nursing and Midwifery Council (2018a) Future Nurse: The Standards of Proficiency for Registered Nurses. https://www.nmc.org.uk/globalassets/sitedocuments/education-standards/future-nurse-proficiencies.pdf (last accessed December 2020).

The annexes

There are two annexes to the standards of proficiency. They provide a description of what registered nurses should be able to demonstrate they can do at the point of registration in order to provide safe nursing care. In Annexe A, the communication and relationship management skills required are detailed. Annexe B specifies the nursing procedures that registered nurses must demonstrate that they are able to perform safely are described. As with the knowledge proficiencies, the annexes have identified where more advanced skills are required by registered nurses, working in a specific field of nursing practice.

> ## Over to you
>
> Registered nurses in all fields of nursing practice are required to demonstrate the ability to communicate and manage relationships with a range of people, people of all ages with a range of mental, physical, cognitive and behavioural health challenges. Think about how you would have to adapt your practices to ensure that the various groups of people have their needs met.

Annexe A

The communication and relationship management skills that a newly registered nurse must be able to demonstrate has to meet the proficiency outcomes that are outlined in the standards, these skills are set out in Annexe A. Key to the provision of safe and compassionate person-centred care is effective communication. Registered nurses in all fields of nursing practice must be able to demonstrate the ability to communicate and manage relationships with people of all ages with a range of mental, physical, cognitive and behavioural health challenges. Practising in a diverse range of environments with a variety of people requires a broad spectrum of communication and relationship management skills which can help to ensure that individuals, their families and carers are a part of and understand care decisions. These skills are important when undertaking an accurate and culturally aware assessment of care needs, making sure that the needs, priorities, expertise and preferences of people will be valued and taken into consideration. If a person has special communication needs or they have a disability, reasonable adjustments must be implemented to communicate, provide and share information in such a way that the adjustments will encourage understanding and engagement as well as enabling equal access care of a high quality. Four sections within Annexe A set out the communication and relationship management skills. At the point of registration, the registered nurse will be able to safely demonstrate the following skills:

- Underpinning communication skills for assessing, planning, providing and managing best practice, evidence-based nursing care.

- Evidence-based, best-practice approaches to communication for supporting people of all ages, their families and carers in preventing ill health and in managing their care.
- Evidence-based, best-practice communication skills and approaches for providing therapeutic interventions.
- Evidence-based, best-practice communication skills and approaches for working with people in professional teams.

Annexe B

In Annexe B of the standards (NMC 2018a), the nursing procedures required by a newly registered nurse to meet the proficiency outcomes are set out in this annexe. The registered nurse has to be able to undertake these procedures in an effective way in order to offer people compassionate, evidence-based person-centred nursing care. All nursing procedures are to be carried out in such a way that they reflect cultural awareness, ensuring that the needs, priorities, expertise and preferences of people are respected and given consideration. It is essential that a holistic approach to the care of people is adopted.

Regardless of the field of practice, registered nurses have to demonstrate an ability to provide nursing intervention and support for people of all ages who are in need of nursing procedures while the processes of assessment is being undertaken, a diagnosis is being made, care and treatment for mental, physical, cognitive and behavioural health challenges are being provided. Reasonable adjustments are made to ensure that all procedures are undertaken safely. The nursing procedures within Annexe B are set out in two sections.

- Part 1: Procedures for assessing people's needs for person-centred care.
- Part 2: Procedures for the planning, provision and management of person-centred nursing care.

The requirements within the two sections (parts 1 and 2) are applicable to all fields of nursing practice, it is recognised, however, that various care settings may require different approaches to care provision. The NMC expected that the procedures in Annexe B would be assessed in the student's chosen field of practice where this is practicable. At the point of registration, the registered nurse will be able to safely demonstrate the procedures identified in Table 2.4.

TABLE **2.4**

Annexes A and B.

Outcome	Examples of components
Part 1: Procedures for assessing people's needs for person-centred care	
Use evidence-based, best practice approaches to take a history, observe, recognise and accurately assess people of all ages	Mental health and wellbeing status: • signs of mental and emotional distress or vulnerability • cognitive health status and wellbeing • signs of cognitive distress and impairment • behavioural distress based needs • signs of mental and emotional distress including agitation, aggression and challenging behaviour • signs of self-harm and/or suicidal ideation Physical health and wellbeing: • symptoms and signs of physical ill health • symptoms and signs of physical distress symptoms and signs of deterioration and sepsis
Use evidence-based, best practice approaches to undertake the following procedures	• take, record and interpret vital signs • undertake venepuncture, cannulation and blood sampling, interpreting normal and common abnormal blood profiles and venous blood gases • manage routine ECG investigations, interpret normal and commonly encountered abnormal traces • manage blood component transfusions • manage and interpret cardiac monitors, infusion pumps, blood glucose monitors and other monitoring devices • accurately measure weight and height, calculate body mass index, recognise healthy ranges • undertake a whole-body systems assessment • undertake chest auscultation, interpret findings • collect and observe specimens, interpreting findings • measure and interpret blood glucose levels • recognise and respond to signs of all forms of abuse • undertake, respond to and interpret neurological observations and assessments identify and respond to signs of deterioration and sepsis

(Continued)

TABLE **2.4**

(Continued)

Outcome	Examples of components
	• administer basic mental health and physical first aid • recognise and manage seizures, choking and anaphylaxis, provide appropriate basic life support • recognise and respond to challenging behaviour, provide appropriate safe holding and restraint
Part 2: Procedures for the planning, provision and management of person-centred nursing care	
Use evidence-based, best practice approaches for meeting needs for care and support with rest, sleep, comfort and the maintenance of dignity, accurately assessing the person's capacity for independence and self-care and initiating appropriate interventions	• observe and assess comfort, pain and sleep • use appropriate bedmaking techniques and positioning and pressure-relieving techniques • take action to ensure privacy and dignity • take appropriate action to reduce or minimise pain or discomfort • take appropriate action to reduce fatigue, minimise insomnia and support improved rest and sleep hygiene.
Use evidence-based, best practice approaches for meeting the needs for care and support with hygiene and the maintenance of skin integrity, accurately assessing the person's capacity for independence and self-care and initiating appropriate interventions	• observe, assess and optimise skin and hygiene status, determine need for support and intervention • assess skin integrity, use appropriate products to prevent or manage skin breakdown • assess and provide assistance with washing, bathing, shaving and dressing • identify and manage skin irritations and rashes • assess and provide oral, dental, eye and nail care and make onward referral if needed • use aseptic techniques with wound care • assess, respond and manage pyrexia and hypothermia

> **TABLE 2.4**
>
> **(Continued)**

Outcome	Examples of components
Use evidence-based, best practice approaches for meeting needs for care and support with nutrition and hydration, accurately assessing the person's capacity for independence and self-care and initiating appropriate interventions	• observe, assess and optimise nutrition and hydration status • use nutritional assessment tools • assist with feeding and drinking, use appropriate aids • record fluid intake and output, manage dehydration or fluid retention • identify, respond to and manage nausea and vomiting • insert, manage and remove oral/nasal/gastric tubes • manage artificial nutrition and hydration using various routes • manage administration of intravenous fluids • manage fluid and nutritional infusion pumps and devices
Use evidence-based, best practice approaches for meeting needs for care and support with bladder and bowel health, accurately assessing the person's capacity for independence and self-care and initiating appropriate interventions	• assess urinary and bowel continence, determine need for support and intervention, assist with toileting, manage use of appropriate aids • use appropriate continence products • insert, manage and remove catheters (all genders), assist with self-catheterisation • manage bladder drainage • assess bladder and bowel patterns, identify and respond to constipation, diarrhoea and urinary and faecal retention • administer enemas and suppositories, undertake rectal examination and manual evacuation when appropriate • undertake stoma care identify and use appropriate products and approaches.
Use evidence-based, best practice approaches for meeting needs for care and support with mobility and safety, accurately assessing the person's capacity for independence and self-care and initiating appropriate interventions	• use evidence-based risk assessment tools to determine need for support and intervention to optimise mobility and safety, identify and manage risk of falls • use contemporary moving and handling techniques and mobility aids • use moving and handling equipment, supporting people with impaired mobility • use appropriate safety techniques and devices

(Continued)

TABLE **2.4**

(Continued)

Outcome	Examples of components
Use evidence-based, best practice approaches for meeting needs for respiratory care and support, accurately assessing the person's capacity for independence and self-care and initiating appropriate interventions	• assess need for intervention and respond to restlessness, agitation and breathlessness • manage administration of oxygen using a range of routes and best-practice approaches • take and interpret peak flow and oximetry measurements • use nasal and oral suctioning techniques • manage inhalation, humidifier and nebuliser devices • manage airway and respiratory processes and equipment
Use evidence-based, best practice approaches for meeting needs for care and support with the prevention and management of infection, accurately assessing the person's capacity for independence and self-care and initiating appropriate interventions	• assess and respond rapidly to potential infection risks using best practice guidelines • use standard precautions protocols • use effective aseptic, non-touch techniques • use appropriate personal protection equipment • implement isolation procedures • use evidence-based hand hygiene techniques • safely decontaminate equipment and environment • safely use and dispose of waste, laundry and sharps • safely assess and manage invasive medical devices and lines
Use evidence-based, best practice approaches for meeting needs for care and support at the end of life, accurately assessing the person's capacity for independence and selfcare and initiating appropriate interventions	• assess the need for intervention for people, families and carers, identify, assess, respond appropriately to uncontrolled symptoms and signs of distress • manage and monitor effectiveness of symptom relief medication, infusion pumps and other devices • assess and review preferences and care priorities of the dying person and their family and carer • understand and apply organ and tissue donation protocols, advanced planning decisions, living wills and health and lasting powers of attorney for health

TABLE 2.4
(Continued)

Outcome	Examples of components
	• understand and apply DNACPR (do not attempt cardiopulmonary resuscitation) decisions and verification of expected death • provide care for the deceased person and the bereaved
Procedural competencies required for best practice, evidence-based medicines administration and optimisation	• undertake initial and continued assessments of people receiving care and ability to self-administer own medications • recognise various procedural routes under which medicines can be prescribed, supplied, dispensed and administered; and the laws, policies, regulations and guidance underpinning them • use the principles of safe remote prescribing and directions to administer medicines • undertake accurate drug calculations • undertake accurate checks, including transcription and titration, of any direction to supply or administer a medicinal product • exercise professional accountability in ensuring the safe administration of medicines • administer injections using intramuscular, subcutaneous, intradermal and intravenous routes, manage injection equipment • administer medications using a range of routes • administer and monitor medications using vascular access devices and enteral equipment • recognise and respond to adverse or abnormal reactions to medications • undertake safe storage, transportation and disposal of medicinal products

DNACPR, do not attempt cardiopulmonary resuscitation; ECG, electrocardiogram.
Source: Adapted from NMC (2018a).

How to

In Annexe B (part 1), you have to be able to demonstrate your ability to collect and observe sputum, urine and stool specimens, undertaking routine analysis and interpreting findings.

How would you assess, monitor and record urine?

A urine specimen can be analysed using a number of different tests. These tests can help diagnose certain diseases, monitor their progress, for the purpose of screening in health. They permit laboratory culture to identify pathogenic micro-organisms and determine drug sensitivity. The nurse needs to observe, communicate and measure in order assess effectively.

Infection control protocols must be instigated prior to assessing, monitoring and recording urine. Ensure that all equipment used is safe and leak proof specimen containers are used.

Standard precautions must be followed: all cuts and abrasions must be covered with waterproof dressings. Wear gloves when in contact with body fluids, if there is a risk of splash, face protection must be worn. Wash hands before and after procedure. All spillages of body fluids must be decontaminated appropriately.

Urinalysis

Testing urine involves assessing the elements of the urine by observational, biochemical and mechanical method. Urine testing does not require an aseptic technique, all equipment should be clean and disposable.

Observations

Odour: Fresh urine from a healthy individual should not have an offensive odour, but decomposing urine smells like ammonia. A patient whose urine is found to have a 'sweet' smell may be investigated further for diabetes mellitus. Urine smelling of fish can be an indication of infection of the urinary system.

Colour: The normal colour of urine ranges from pale straw to dark amber and varies according to the amount of fluid that has been taken into the body. The type and amount of urinary constituents also affects the colour of urine; dark-coloured urine can, for example, be an indication of dehydration or the presence of bile pigments, a manifestation of liver or biliary tract disease. Certain food and drugs alter the colour of a patient's urine: beetroot can cause the urine to take on an orange-red hue.

Haematuria: The term to describe blood in the urine. This can vary from microscopic haematuria (i.e. that is detected only by testing) to frank haematuria, with an obvious red colouration. Blood in the urine is suggestive of disease or damage to the renal system.

Glycosuria: This presence of glucose in the urine, which can be suggestive of diabetes mellitus.

Proteinuria: This term used when there is protein in the urine, which can be a manifestation of acute or chronic renal disease.

Ketones: Ketones are produced when the body metabolises fat; ketones are one of the products of this metabolism. Ketones are acidotic, so if the excessive metabolism of fat persists, a state of metabolic acidosis develops, which can, if untreated, lead to coma and death. At a certain stage of acidosis, the ketones are excreted by the urinary system they may be indicative of excessive fasting or uncontrolled or poorly controlled diabetes mellitus.

Nitrites: This test relies on the breakdown of urinary nitrates to nitrites, which are not found in normal urine. Many Gram-negative and some Gram-positive bacteria are capable of producing this reaction and a positive test suggests their presence in significant numbers. A negative result does not rule out a urinary tract infection.

Leucocytes: A positive result suggests pyuria (pus in the urine) associated with urinary tract infection.

Specific gravity: Varies with the state of hydration.

pH: The pH of urine reflects the function of the kidney in maintaining the acid–base balance.

Equipment

- Clean dry bowl, bedpan or urinal
- Reagent strips (check expiry date prior to using)
- Watch with a second hand
- Gloves

Procedure

- Read reagent strip manufacture's guidelines.
- The privacy and dignity of the patient should be maintained throughout the procedure.
- Explain procedure and obtain consent from patient.

- Perform hand hygiene.
- Gloves must be applied.
- Request patient to pass urine into container (assist if necessary).
- Observe, report and record urine for sediment, colour and odour.
- Remove reagent strip ensuring you do not touch the reagent squares as this may contaminate strips.
- Immerse the strip fully in urine.
- Withdraw the strip from the urine and gently tap on the rim of the container to remove the excess.
- Hold the strip at an angle to prevent cross contamination from one reagent pad to another.
- Hold the strip vertically or horizontally against the results guidance chart to ensure an accurate interpretation of the colour change.
- Read the reagent strip after the recommended time has elapsed to ensure accurate results.
- Dispose of the excess urine into the toilet bowl.
- Dispose of equipment (adhere to local policy and procedure).
- Hand hygiene must be carried out after procedure.
- All results should be reported and documented, note the results providing an accurate written record.
- The patient should be reassured regarding the results.

Source: Adapted from Bardsley (2015).

Consider also how you would:

- Recognise when a urine specimen would be required.
- Identify the equipment required to take a catheter specimen of urine.
- Ensure that you are adhering to local policy in obtaining a catheter specimen of urine.
- Store and transport a urine specimen in accordance with local policy.
- Document and report your activities and any findings.

The standards for student supervision and assessment

These standards set out the NMC's requirements for the learning, support and supervision of students in the practice environment. They also set out how students are assessed for theory and practice learning.

Students are supported within the place of their learning placement by designated practice supervisors and a range of registered and non-registered health and social care professionals throughout the nursing programme. The standards for student supervision and assessment (NMC 2018c) replaced the NMCs (2008) standards to support learning and assessment in practice.

Chapter 8 of this text considers the standards for student supervision and assessment in detail. In that chapter, an overview of the standards is provided, together with a discussion of the learning environments, various roles and responsibilities, and practical advice concerning student supervision and assessment.

Complete this activity now

This chapter has provided much detail about the skills you are required to learn to demonstrate proficiency at the end of your three-year programme of study and prior to admission to the register. Look at Table 2.4 and see if you can match the content to the 12 activities of living (Roper et al. 2000).

Activity of living	Content of Annexes A and B
Maintaining a safe environment	
Breathing	
Communication	
Eating and drinking	
Eliminating	
Personal cleansing and dressing	
Controlling body temperature	
Mobilising	
Working and playing	
Expressing sexuality	
Sleeping	
Dying	

Summary

In 2018 the NMC published a range of standards that impact nurse education. This chapter has focussed primarily on the standards of proficiency for registered nurses. It is important to understand how these standards are used in your programme of study. The assessment of clinical skills is detailed in the two annexes that accompany the standards. The content of the annexes are mapped into the practice assessment document ensuring that at the point of registration the nurse is able to demonstrate proficiency across a range of skills with a range of people on a range of care environments.

References

Bardsley, A. (2015). How to perform a urinalysis. *Nursing Standard* 30 (2): 34–36.

Department for Education (2022). Ofsted Inspection and ESFA intervention. www.gov.uk/government/publications/provider-guide-to-delivering-high-quality-apprenticeships/ofsted-inspection-and-esfa-intervention (accessed July 2022).

Education and Skills Funding Agency (2022). Apprenticeship gateway and resits for endpoint assessment EPA. www.gov.uk/guidance/apprenticeship-gateway-and-resits-for-end-point-assessment-epa (accessed July 2022).

House of Commons (2020). Public Accounts Committee NHS Nursing Workforce. Eighteenth Report of Session 2019–21 HC408. https://publications.parliament.uk/pa/cm5801/cmselect/cmpubacc/408/408.pdf (accessed December 2020).

Immonen, K., Oikarainen, A., Tomietto, M. et al. (2019). Assessment of nursing students' competence in clinical practice: a systematic review of reviews. *International Journal of Nursing Studies* 100: 103414. https://doi.org/10.1016/j.ijnurstu.2019.103414.

National Audit Office (2020). The NHS Nursing Workforce. HC109. www.nao.org.uk/wp-content/uploads/2020/03/The-NHS-nursing-workforce.pdf (accessed December 2020).

NHS England (2019). The NHS Long Term Plan. www.longtermplan.nhs.uk/wp-content/uploads/2019/08/nhs-long-term-plan-version-1.2.pdf (accessed December 2020)

Nursing and Midwifery Council (2008). *Standards to Support Learning and Assessment in Practice*. London: NMC.

Nursing and Midwifery Council (2018a). Future Nurse: The Standards of Proficiency for Registered Nurses. www.nmc.org.uk/globalassets/sitedocuments/education-standards/future-nurse-proficiencies.pdf (accessed December 2020)

Nursing and Midwifery Council (2018b). Standards of Proficiency for Registered Nursing Associates. www.nmc.org.uk/standards/standards-for-nursing-associates/standards-of-proficiency-for-nursing-associates (accessed March 2023).

Nursing and Midwifery Council (2018c). The Standards for Student Supervision and Assessment. www.nmc.org.uk/standards-for-education-and-training/standards-for-student-supervision-and-assessment (accessed December 2020)

Roper, N., Logan, W., and Tierney, A. (2000). *The Roper Logan Tierney Model of Nursing.* Edinburgh: Churchill Livingstone.

CHAPTER 3

Learning to learn

Luke Cox

AIM

This chapter encourages the reader to begin understanding how learning works, to explore some of the methods that universities and other education institutions may use to promote active learning, and to begin considering the role of the student as a self-directed learner.

LEARNING OUTCOMES

Having read this chapter, the reader will:

1. Appreciate learning as an active process.
2. Understand simulation and 'the flipped classroom' as learning methods.
3. Be able to begin developing a strategy to become a self-directed learner.

Introduction

You have made an important decision to study nursing. It is a big step, and you are committing yourself to years of study in theory and practice. Nursing is undoubtedly a rewarding profession, and many people will benefit from your care and support. Nursing can also be mentally challenging and physically exhausting. You may work long, unsocial hours in stressful, unpredictable and emotional circumstances. Your ability to manage this depends to a great extent on your growth as a professional.

You will need to 'learn how to learn' from your successes, and also from times when things have not gone so well. You must reflect on your practice and keep on top of new developments in your chosen field. These are not just suggestions, these are requirements within the standards of the profession: the Nursing and Midwifery Council (NMC) 'Code' (NMC 2018). Throughout your career as a nurse, you will be regularly called upon to show evidence that this process of learning and development is continuing. Being able to be involved in and responsible for your own learning from the outset will help you immensely on your chosen career path.

Over to you

Take some time to think of the various ways in which you might ensure that you are on top of new developments in your chosen field.

Go online

Revalidation is the process that all nurses and midwives in the UK and nursing associates in England must follow to maintain their registration with the NMC. Revalidation helps registrants to develop and reflect on their practice and is required every three years. The NMC has produced standards regarding revalidation. Take a look at the NMC website:

www.nmc.org.uk/revalidation

where there is a range of resources for registrants associated with revalidation. The resources may be of value to you in a number of ways.

Those around you will want you to succeed in your studies and will want to help you learn. While you are at university, the academic and skills curriculum will have been designed with maximising your learning opportunities in mind, and it is likely that the methods employed will be different to those you are used to. Understanding the thinking behind those processes will help you make the most of the opportunities presented.

Green flag

It is important that you make use of the various resources that are available to you in practice and in the university setting. If you need guidance, always speak to those who are supervising or supporting you. Resources can be human and material.

This chapter emphasises the need to 'learn how to learn'. This means developing strategies that will help you get the most out of learning. Understanding why teaching might be structured or delivered in a particular way will assist with this process. It is important to appreciate that learning is most effective when it is a process in which you play a central and active role. Box 3.1 provides some key words around learning.

Hear it from the student

When I started my nursing degree, I was so surprised at the many different approaches used to teach me. Importantly, it not just how they teach you but how you learn, so much of the emphasis is on you, the learner. I love the different methods that are used at uni but, beware, they can take you by surprise and they all take some getting used to – especially the role play!

Daniel, second-year learning disabilities student

Box 3.1 | Key words in learning

Active learning: A learning method in which students are involved in the teaching and learning process.
Blended learning: A learning method in which self-directed tasks, often with online components, complement more traditional classroom-based teaching methods.

Bloom's taxonomy: A way of describing the aims of teaching in terms of the expectations of learner achievement.

Constructivism: A theory of learning which suggests learners are active in creating their own knowledge and understanding of reality.

Curriculum: (plural curricula) The range subjects taught and learned to complete a course, or part of a course, in UK nursing mapped against NMC requirements for education and registration as a nurse.

Debriefing: A structured method of reflection following a clinical incident or (in an educational context) a simulation exercise.

Experiential learning: An educational theory developed by David Kolb, an American educationalist, which suggests learning is a cycle of active experimentation and reflection.

Flipped classroom: A type of blended learning in which traditional classroom activities are moved to online or pre-reading activities, and face-to-face sessions are used for activities based around problem solving or using skills in context

Forum theatre: A type of performance in which actors and audience are all participants and can engage with one another. This may be used as a type of clinical simulation.

Immersive technology: Technology which allows a participant to be engaged in simulated environments, for instance virtual reality or 'high-fidelity' simulation.

Learning style: A theory that individuals have a preferred way of learning and that teaching can be adapted to meet the requirements of that style.

Manikin: Sometimes written as 'mannequin' and also referred to as a *human patient simulator*. This is a robot which can replicate some of the features of a human patient or service user, particularly in terms of physiological characteristics such as pulse and blood pressure, and is often used in clinical simulation.

Metacognition: Literally 'thinking about thinking – the idea that thinking about your thought process (for instance in term of how you learn) will help you adjust and improve your performance.

Non-technical skills/human factors: Often used interchangeably, these terms often appear in studies of human error; they suggest that performance may be dependent on communication, the environment and how systems are designed, not just individual competence in a skill or procedure.

OSCE: An objective structured clinical examination, an assessment method used in many clinical disciplines including nursing and medicine to assess skills, often consisting of an assessment of an actor or manikin playing a patient role.

Passive learning: Often called 'direct instruction', a method of teaching and learning where the learner receives and internalises information without feedback. A lecture is a typically example of a passive learning experience.

Reflection: A way of making sense of experienced events, which derives from experiential learning theory and is seen as an important skill in a nurse's professional development.

Role play: A type of peer-to-peer teaching in which students take on the roles of a patient, relative or another health care professional to practise interpersonal communication and skills.

Simulation: A teaching methodology in which the environment and events of a clinical setting are recreated to practise skills and consider associated human factors, usually combined with debriefing.

Virtual/augmented reality: Types of immersive technology where entire environments are recreated for instance within a viewing headset (in virtual reality) or where technology is used to recreate some elements of a clinical environment (augmented reality).

Active and passive learning

Active learning is based on a theory of education called constructivism. The central idea behind this theory is that learners develop understanding of the world through interacting with it, as opposed to knowledge consisting in objective, unalterable facts. In this sense, learning is a process of 'making meaning'. Deeper levels of understanding are achieved by analysing, evaluating and synthesising ideas.

You may believe that there is a particular way in which you learn best, and you may at some point complete a questionnaire or survey that seeks to classify your individual 'learning style' – identifying for instance that you are a 'visual' or 'kinaesthetic' learner. This may not be a helpful way for you to think about learning and is not well supported by the evidence we have about how people learn. The context of nursing education is of striking a balance between theory and practice, which is best achieved by exposing you to varied learning experiences. A more realistic theory in education is that students learn most effectively when they can see the usefulness of what they are learning and the meaningful connections between theory and practice in the real world.

Over to you

What are the principles associated with constructivism?
What do you understand by:

• Problem-based learning
• Inquiry-based learning

When an active learning approach is used, learning is not only about the content. It is also about the process. Active learning develops students' autonomy and their ability to be self-directed in learning. Nurses are required to become autonomous practitioners and, to do this, you will need greater involvement and control over your learning. This in turn will enable you to continue learning once you graduate and participate in lifelong learning – and again this is a requirement of nursing as a profession.

Green flag

Being active in your learning will prepare you for the role you that will play as a registered nurse.

Active learning contrasts with passive learning, in which learners are the recipients of information. A passive learner can build an impressive knowledge base by rote but may not be able to establish connections between different areas of that knowledge or employ that knowledge with autonomy in practical situations. An example of a passive learning experience would be sitting in a lecture theatre, or an online lecture, watching a presentation without feedback or interaction. Knowledge is certainly important, and the need for active learning does not mean that lecturers will not play a part in your education, but remembering information is only of value if it can be part of an application in context. Knowing that haloperidol is a medicine that is used to manage symptoms of schizophrenia is useful but exploring the social context of why someone may have stopped taking this medication as prescribed and involving them in a person-centred solution requires a set of competencies beyond merely receiving and remembering knowledge.

A theoretical perspective which guides how education is structured to achieve these 'higher' competencies is Bloom's taxonomy (Figure 3.1), named after American educational psychologist Benjamin Bloom and since revised and updated (Anderson et al. 2001). Learners can build on knowledge to develop comprehension and understanding, before applying their understanding in novel, practical situations, developing new ideas of their own and evaluating different ideas. Because this is part of a popular and accessible theory in education, universities are likely to design their curricula with Bloom's taxonomy in mind, with the aim of reaching higher levels in this structure.

As a nurse, developing evaluative and analytical skills will help you to become more proficient at problem solving, decision making, and applying your knowledge. As a learner, it will be helpful for you to evaluate each learning task you undertake before you begin them. Is the aim of the task for you to remember a list of facts or are you being asked to make connections between those facts and their context, or to weigh up different perspectives? A clue will be in the sorts of words which are used to describe tasks and assessments, so be on the lookout

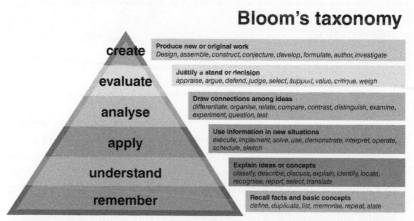

Bloom's taxonomy

create
Produce new or original work
Design, assemble, construct, conjecture, develop, formulate, author, investigate

evaluate
Justify a stand or decision
appraise, argue, defend, judge, select, support, value, critique, weigh

analyse
Draw connections among ideas
differentiate, organise, relate, compare, contrast, distinguish, examine, experiment, question, test

apply
Use information in new situations
execute, implement, solve, use, demonstrate, interpret, operate, schedule, sketch

understand
Explain ideas or concepts
classify, describe, discuss, explain, identify, locate, recognise, report, select, translate

remember
Recall facts and basic concepts
define, duplicate, list, memorise, repeat, state

FIGURE 3.1 Bloom's taxonomy. *Source:* Vanderbilt University, Center for Teaching (https://cft.vanderbilt.edu/guides-sub-pages/blooms-taxonomy).

for verbs from Bloom's taxonomy when evaluating the tasks you are set. An assignment asking you to 'compare and contrast' two different nursing theories will require you to organise your thinking in a different way from a task where you are describing the function of an organ in the body.

Write here

In the list below, think of some verbs related to Bloom's taxonomy that you could use in tasks and assessments.

Bloom's taxonomy	Suggested verbs
Remember: • Recognising • Recalling	
Understand: • Interpreting • Exemplifying • Classifying • Summarising • Inferring • Comparing • Explaining	
Apply: • Executing • Implementing	
Analyse: • Differentiating • Organising • Attributing	
Evaluate: • Checking • Critiquing	
Create: • Generating • Planning • Producing	

To help to illustrate the difference between active and passive learning, and the idea that there may be different levels to learning, consider how you might learn how to bake a cake. It would be straightforward to remember a shopping list for cake making, together with a series of steps for blending and cooking these ingredients. You could understand the properties of different flours and raising agents and learn recipes for several different types of cake in this way. Then, after a period of revision, you could sit an exam about cake making. Suppose you passed this exam with a distinction. Would this mean that you could actually bake a cake? You might argue that a cake-making course in which you experiment with mixing ingredients, using different sorts of flours and spatulas, and different temperatures and cooking times, and in which people observe this process and taste your cakes and offer feedback, might better equip you for making cakes in the real world. You would know what techniques work for you and the process would result in a tasty cake. It may be that not every cake you make in this process would be a success, and this might be a more expensive way to learn in terms of the time you spend and the resources you use. But you would learn how to solve problems and substitute ingredients where necessary, and you would be better placed to be innovative, perhaps creating your own methods and recipes.

Within nursing education, an active learning approach means structuring teaching and learning so that you are given opportunities to construct your own meaning, by exploring your theoretical knowledge of concepts within practical, real-world contexts. Of course, your clinical placements will provide you with fantastic opportunities to contextualise knowledge, but you are also likely to find your academic studies involve techniques such as role play, group discussions, concept mapping, forum theatre, and even the use of immersive technology such as virtual reality. The use of a combination of online and classroom-based activities is often referred to as blended learning and is likely to be a characteristic of your nursing education. This approach places more emphasis on your own learning as you will have tasks to complete outside of the classroom setting. This chapter considers specific examples of active learning techniques in more depth, in exploring flipped classroom approaches to learning and the use of simulation as a teaching and learning method.

Active learning: the flipped classroom

'The flipped classroom' is an approach in teaching that you are likely to experience at university. It is a type of blended learning in which face-to-face teaching sessions are complemented by self-directed activities and online learning. The flipped classroom is an extension of the principle in which the activities that might traditionally be seen as 'homework' or a follow-up to a teaching session are brought within the classroom, while emphasis is placed on preparatory study *before* a face-to-face session. Classroom sessions then become an opportunity to explore, apply and contextualise this newly acquired knowledge. As a structure, this can work particularly effectively for teaching practical skills, as students can come to classroom skills sessions already equipped with underlying theoretical knowledge. You might find that online teaching aids (e.g. platforms such as Moodle, Canvas or Blackboard) are populated with learning opportunities related to forthcoming face-to-face sessions, with formative assessments to test your knowledge and understanding of underlying concepts.

Hear it from the student

I started my nursing education after a career change, so I am what is known as a 'mature student'. I was so very bewildered with all the technology that we were expected to use, online teaching, e-learning and so on. Truly, this was a mountain for me to climb, and I really struggled. As time went on, though, I became more confident and competent in using the various technologies. I asked people for help, including my family, the librarians and technical support staff at uni were just so patient with me and eventually I mastered it all. Well, I thought I did, but like nursing teaching approaches are in a constant state of change so I have indeed become a lifelong learner.

Maureen, third-year adult nursing student

As an example, it is likely that you will learn how to record someone's blood pressure using a stethoscope and sphygmomanometer. This is a fundamental skill, if not an easy one. Teaching you to do this procedure could consist of a lecture, in which the anatomy of the arteries in the body is discussed, and the physiology of the circulatory system, alongside the reasons why blood pressure is a meaningful observation to record and the implications of a blood pressure reading outside a normal range, before moving to a demonstration of the procedure, and then some time for you to practise this skill.

Alternatively, in the flipped classroom, you could watch recorded demonstrations of the procedure online and study skills guides, conduct preparatory reading about anatomy and physiology, supported perhaps by self-assessments, and do this all *before* the face-to-face session, which would provide you with longer to familiarise yourself with the equipment, practice the skill itself, and to contextualise the skill within a scenario – for instance using role play or simulation.

The challenge you might find with this second version of the blood pressure session is in managing your time and being able to be a self-directed learner when away from the classroom setting, particularly if this is an unfamiliar way of learning. If you have not engaged in relevant pre-reading, study and assessment then the classroom session could be baffling and without context. What we know from studies of students taught this way is that they value this structure of teaching highly, but that it can initially feel threatening. Understanding why this structure is being used, and being prepared to engage with it, will be of great benefit to you, but it will require you to be able to learn autonomously outside the classroom setting. Box 3.2 provides some tips that might help you get the most out of blended learning approaches in general and flipped classroom teaching particularly.

Box 3.2 | Tips for students using blended learning

Be information technology ready

There may be computer-based and online tasks as part of any blended learning approach. Check that you can access websites before you need them, especially if they are sites external to the university requiring a login and password.

Get training and seek support

Not everyone is used to using computers to work, research and write. Seek help from your university library if you feel that you need additional support, training on a new computer platform or access to information technology (IT) equipment. Some universities will offer support in purchasing computers for home use and most will have contracts with organisations to provide software (for instance check if you can download Microsoft Office 365 for free at home under the university's licence).

Read ahead and plan ahead

Look at tasks set for forthcoming weeks and use a diary or online calendar to plan your own sessions to go through pre-reading related to upcoming face-to-face sessions.

Assess the learning

Consider carefully what you are being asked to do before a session. If you are watching a video or a recorded lecture, what questions are you being asked to consider? What resources will you need to access?

Engage in face-to-face learning

Classroom sessions will be a chance to contextualise learning you have started elsewhere. Be prepared to engage with activities and practice skills.

Collaborate

Classroom sessions may involve group work and discussions. Be respectful of the contributions of others and explore other perspectives on the same tasks.

Reflect

Consider how the process of a different learning method has made you feel. What worked well about the way you set yourself up to prepare for the session? Did you feel that you had done enough to be an engaged participant? Consider what you might do differently the next time.

Active learning: simulation

Simulation is used by many universities during nursing courses as a method of teaching, learning and, sometimes, assessment. It is also used extensively in clinical settings as a way of developing staff teams.

Most universities will have a simulation centre that replicates experiences you might find in a clinical setting or in a patient or service user's home.

Often, simulation centres are technologically advanced, with genuine clinical equipment, cameras to film activity and human patient simulators (or 'manikins'). For a new student, this environment can be daunting, so understanding the reasons for employing simulation as a learning method may be helpful. A key reason for using simulation is to help consolidate skills and understanding within a safe space, perhaps carrying out a risky task but with the element of risk removed.

A supervisor's notes

I often take part in assisting with simulation at our local university, where I will work with students who are allocated to our GP practice. While simulation is not hands-on clinical practice, it can be the closest thing to it.

Our GP practice is so busy that teaching new clinical skills to our students can sometimes be a challenge. What is really helpful is knowing that students have been using simulation at university and, as such, they will have the mastered the fundamental aspects of the various complex skills. Knowing this and assessing a student in practice on the 'shop floor' real makes a big difference. The student is much more confident and less hesitant to undertake a supervised skill if they have some simulated input.

Renuka, general practice nurse

As an example, you may be able to calculate the required amount of a particular medication competently in the quiet of a classroom. It may be more difficult to do the same within a stressful environment, with alarms sounding and a confused and scared patient crying out in pain, all of which can be replicated during a simulated scenario. Exploring the 'non-technical skills' or 'human factors' that influence our ability to perform skills is often an aim of learning using simulation. This derives from the use of simulation to improve safety in other 'high risk' industries, such as aviation or generating nuclear power. As with flight simulators, being able to make mistakes in a controlled environment can help improve your confidence and ultimately the safety of those to whom you will be offering care and support.

Simulation can be used as means of academic assessment, with structured, repeatable scenarios forming the basis of an exam. This may be referred to as an objective structured clinical examination (OSCE). You may also find that simulated clinical situations are used to assess your competency in particular skills that are contained within pre-registration standards but to which you have not been exposed during clinical placements (i.e. a competency within your practice assessment document).

Complete this activity now

Make a list of the skills you have been taught using simulation and then match them to the skills that you have achieve as part of assessment in clinical practice.

Skills taught in simulation	Skills that need to be completed in clinical practice

Simulation is also likely to be used by universities as a means of adding to or replacing the hours you spend in clinical practice. At the time of writing, in the UK the NMC allows each student to spend up to 300 hours in simulated practice experiences instead of in clinical placement across the duration of their course, with some universities permitted to use up to 600 hours in this manner (NMC 2022). This can help universities and students where there are challenges with accessing placements, where unusual events create restrictions (as with the COVID-19 pandemic) or to provide an experience that the student might not otherwise gain (for instance a mental health nursing setting for a student studying a different field of nursing). There is evidence to support this approach, and it is likely that a 'virtual placement' will form a part of your clinical education.

Try this in practice

When next in practice, think about the clinical skills you are performing. Were any of these skills initially taught to you though simulation? What are the pros and cons of simulation?

While approaches to simulation will vary between universities, simulation is generally used as a tool to promote reflection. This might be encouraged by using a structured debriefing method, such as 'PEARLS' or the 'diamond'. Further reading is suggested at the end of the chapter through which you can explore these debriefing models.

Complete this activity now

What does the acronym PEARLS mean:

	Meaning
P	
E	
A	
R	
L	
S	

Go online

Here is a link to the Diamond, a structure for simulation debrief (Jaye et al. 2015):

www.fhft.nhs.uk/media/2699/06_the-diamond-structure-for-simulation-debreif_jaye-et-al.pdf

Take a look at this publication; note the two figures used in paper that highlight the features associated with debriefing using the Diamond model.

You will quickly learn that reflection will play an important role in your development as nurse. You will be encouraged in practice to reflect on events and this will form a key feature of lifelong learning beyond your time as a pre-registration student. A reflective process is a way of breaking down events so they are described and then analysed, with the goal of making a plan for future action so you can develop your practice in response. A commonly applied cycle for reflection is that developed by Graham Gibbs (1998), shown in Figure 3.2, which is based on a theory of education called experiential learning; simply put, the idea that we 'learn by doing'.

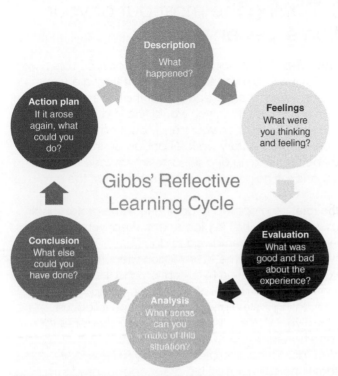

FIGURE 3.2 Gibbs' reflective learning cycle.

The evidence for using simulation as a teaching method is not conclusive, in the sense that it is difficult to demonstrate that using it makes patients safer or happier. However, simulation does tend to be highly valued by students as a means of improving their confidence. There is support for the idea that simulation can effectively replace some clinical placement hours (Hayden et al. 2014), and an expansion of the number hours universities can use simulation in as part of your education is a future possibility. As with all active learning methods, the aim is to place you at the centre of the learning and so getting the most from simulation will require some effort on your part. Box 3.3 shows some tips that might help make your simulation experiences more rewarding.

Becoming a self-directed learner

From the examples of learning methods such as the flipped classroom and simulation, you can see that there is much you can do yourself to become a central participant in your learning; without your involvement

Box 3.3 | Getting the most out of your simulation experiences

- **Suspend your disbelief:** clinical simulation experiences are not real life but it will help you to imagine that they are. Ignore limitations (for instance equipment that does not work properly or is not like the thing you would find in a clinical setting) and focus instead on your behaviour and emotions.
- **Read up:** look at preparatory work set ahead of simulation, which may be pre-reading or a self-assessment task. This will be relevant and will help you to get the most out of the experience.
- **Get into the role:** be prepared to act in the same professional manner as you would whilst in placement. Wear your uniform if this is what you have been asked to do.
- **Be you:** avoid trying to 'game' a simulation scenario. There is not generally a 'right' solution to a situation and the focus is more on how you make decisions. Act as you would in real life.
- **Let it out:** debriefing in simulation is a good time to discuss experiences in your life (e.g. in placement). Be prepared to be open and honest about these experiences.
- **Ask:** the staff facilitating simulation are likely to be experienced practitioners. Simulation is a great opportunity to find out more about anything you are unsure about, either from the simulation scenario or your placement experiences.
- **Debrief:** debriefing during simulation is not designed to be threatening and is not an exploration of your knowledge, and it is not a test. Be prepared to engage honestly with debriefing. It may help you to explore in advance the type of debriefing structure used.
- **Respect confidentiality:** if stories about practice are shared, try not to identify individuals and do not discuss other people's experiences outside the simulation setting.
- **Do not judge:** watching others taking part in simulated scenarios often makes you consider what they *should* do differently but this is not often a helpful way to give feedback. Thinking about *why* people act as they do can be more productive in shaping future performance.
- **Reflect:** take some time on your own to consider experiences in simulation and how they will make a difference to future practice. Written reflections can be added to your portfolio to show your continuing professional development.

these types of teaching will not work at all. This means that what you get out of education depends upon your attitude towards learning and your willingness to get involved. But it can be difficult to engage with tasks set for you to complete outside a classroom setting if they seem arbitrary. Now you understand the reasons for your learning being structured in a particular way, the tasks you are set may appear more meaningful. Nonetheless, taking responsibility for your learning is not easy, and many students find the process of effective independent study to be a challenge. Developing a strategy to manage this is a process of metacognition; that is, thinking about your own thinking. Research in this area suggests that there is cycle of processes you go through when effectively learning in a self-directed way (Figure 3.3).

An awareness of these stages is useful for you as a learner because it will help you to anticipate pitfalls and to structure your learning in a more focused way. Within this cycle, a key step is to assess the task, particularly if you have moved from one type of educational structure to another. Strategies that you used effectively at GCSE and A level can still be applied in higher education, but it is more likely that you will be asked to contextualise and apply learning. Earlier, you read about Bloom's taxonomy as a way of describing the level of competency a learning activity is expected to provide you. Ensure that you are reading and evaluating tasks set for you carefully, with the language of this taxonomy in mind, so you can adapt your learning strategy accordingly.

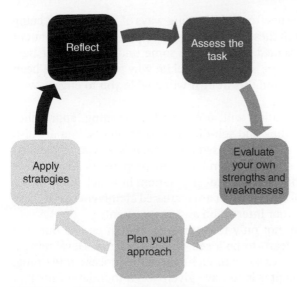

FIGURE 3.3   Cycle of self-directed learning.

Try this in practice

Here are some strategies that might help you as you develop your skills and your practice:

- Break down the task into chunks.
- Be clear about what is being asked of you and what is *not* wanted.
- Rewrite the main goal in your own words and describe the steps you will take to achieve that goal.
- Check the criteria for an assignment; for instance, what the learning outcomes are and the evidence you will need to show you that are meeting them.

Summary

This chapter has explored some theoretical approaches to learning which will be relevant to your studies as a student nurse. Learning is most likely to be effective when it is an active process, particularly in the context of nursing, where the connections you make between theory, practical skills-based elements, and a wider social context will be vital.

You will experience new and challenging ways of learning and being prepared to engage with these methods will help you get the most out of the opportunities presented to you. With some understanding of how learning works you will be able to appreciate why activities have been set up in a certain way, and this in turn will enable you to engage with learning more effectively.

Increasingly, universities will use blended learning approaches where teaching has online and self-directed components. You are also likely to encounter the flipped classroom, which is a type of blended learning where you study independently to prepare for face-to-face sessions. You will experience clinical simulation, in which some of the features of the clinical environment are recreated at university. All these opportunities rely on your interaction and engagement.

An important skill, not only for a pre-registration course but as a lifelong learner, is to learn to be a self-directed learner. Developing a strategy to do this requires some thought about the process of learning, and an aim of this chapter is to have given you a foundation for that understanding.

References

Anderson, L.W., Krathwohl, D.R., Airasian, P.W. et al. (2001). *A Taxonomy for Learning, Teaching, and Assessing: A Revision of Bloom's Taxonomy of Educational Objectives*. New York, NY: Longman.

Gibbs, G. (1998). *Learning by Doing: A Guide to Teaching and Learning Methods*. Oxford: Oxford Brooks University.

Hayden, J., Smiley, R., Alexander, M. et al. (2014). The NCSBN National Simulation Study: a longitudinal, randomized, controlled study replacing clinical hours with simulation in prelicensure nursing education. *Journal of Nursing Regulation* 5: S1–S64. https://doi.org/10.1016/S2155-8256(15)30062-4.

Jaye, P., Thomas, L., and Reedy, G. (2015). The diamond: a structure for simulation debrief. *Clinical Teacher* 12: 171–175. https://doi.org/10.1111/tct.12300.

Nursing and Midwifery Council (2018). *The Code: Professional Standards of Practice and Behaviour for Nurses and Midwives Nursing and Midwifery Council*. London: NMC.

Nursing and Midwifery Council (2022). *Current Recovery Programme Standards*. London: NMC.

Further reading

Ambrose, S., Bridges, M., and Lovett, M. (2010). *How Learning Works: 7 Research-Based Principles for Smart Teaching*. San Francisco, CA: Wiley.

Eppich, W. and Cheng, A. (2015). Promoting Excellence and Reflective Learning in Simulation (PEARLS): development and rationale for a blended approach to health care simulation debriefing. *Simulation in Healthcare* 10 (2): 106–115.

CHAPTER 4

Equality and diversity needs

Sue Jackson, Claire Camara, and Peta Jane Greaves

AIM

This chapter encourages the reader to consider and challenge existing knowledge around equality, diversity and inclusion (EDI), and to take into account the possible impact on the wellbeing of themselves, patients and clients.

LEARNING OUTCOMES

Having read this chapter, readers will:

- Understand the Nursing and Midwifery Council's (NMC) position on EDI.
- Understand the position of academic education institutions on EDI.
- Have an awareness of how unconscious bias may influence culturally sensitive care.
- Be able to appreciate how best to promote EDI for themselves and others.

Succeeding on your Nursing Placement: Supervision, Learning and Assessment for Nursing Students, First Edition. Edited by Ian Peate.

As a student nurse, you will be fortunate enough to work alongside a wide section of society. You will care for people across age ranges (the extent will depend on your field of nursing), and will work with those from a spectrum of gender identities and ethnically diverse backgrounds. Nurses have a duty to promote EDI with those in their care and also with their colleagues. The NMC Code (2018) explicitly states that *everyone* has a right to dignity and respect, and that discrimination of all kinds should be challenged.

First, some brief definitions of EDI:

- Equality: this is about treating people fairly. It does not mean treating all people in the same way. People should not be treated unfairly based characteristics, on aspects such as gender, sex, age or ethnicity.
- Diversity: recognising and valuing individual difference.
- Inclusion: feeling valued and psychologically safe.

Background to equality, diversity and inclusion

Historically, and in some situations today, certain groups in society are not treated fairly. Consequently, they have not experienced healthcare in the same way as others (Royal College of Nursing 2021). This has resulted in unequal, unfair and discriminative practices leading to health inequalities, dissatisfaction with services and, consequently, reluctance to seek help when needed (NMC 2020).

In EDI terms, the notion of 'fairness' is a relatively recent development. For example, male homosexual acts were illegal until the introduction of the Sexual Offences Act 1967. As another example, until the Race Relations Act 1965, there was no law to prevent discrimination on the basis of race. In 1998, the Human Rights Act was introduced to protect everybody's basic human rights regardless of nationality or social status. These rights are based on values such as dignity, fairness, equality, respect, and independence.

The Equality Act, introduced in 2010, replaced nine previous pieces of legislation, each targeting particular forms of discrimination. It attempts to counteract the stigmatisation of individuals who have certain physical characteristics, exhibit particular behaviours, or belong to particular groups (which may or may not be identifiable from their appearance). The Equality Act 2010 protects individuals from unfair treatment based on nine protected characteristics. The protected characteristics are highlighted in Box 4.1.

Box 4.1 | The nine protected character-istics identified in the Equality Act 2010

1. Age
2. Disability
3. Gender reassignment
4. Marriage and civil partnership
5. Pregnancy and maternity
6. Race
7. Religious or beliefs
8. Sex
9. Sexual orientation

Write here

How is disability legally defined?

A person can be affected by inequalities associated with multiple characteristics. This is known as intersectionality. Intersectionality can result in a person having a number of interconnected characteristics leading to possible exposure to many forms of discrimination.

Despite changes to the law, there are still examples of discrimination today. For example, according to Bachmann and Gooch (2018), one in seven people from the lesbian, gay, bisexual, transgender, queer or questioning, intersex, asexual, and more (LBGTQ+) community have avoided seeking treatment for a health issue for fear of discrimination. Some health promotion activity is not considered culturally sensitive, leading to poor uptake and subsequently poorer health outcome for certain groups (Public Health England 2018). Within health and social care, it is therefore imperative that peoples' differences are valued, and that everyone is treated equally (Royal College of Nursing 2021).

Discrimination

Discrimination can be defined as harming someone's rights just because of who they are and what they believe, and this leads to inequity (Amnesty International 2023). While discrimination can be defined with respect to each specific characteristic, in health and social care four broad categories are recognised based on how the discrimination is manifest: direct discrimination, indirect discrimination, discrimination by perception and associative discrimination.

Direct discrimination

Direct discrimination is where an individual or group are treated less favourably because of their protected characteristic(s).

Example

Ryan's epilepsy is well controlled. Despite having established reasonable adjustments in other placements, his new ward is reluctant to have him because they believe that he will need to be observed at all times in case he has a seizure and this will add to their workload.

Indirect discrimination

Indirect discrimination is where a policy or procedure is applied to everyone but it puts those with a particular characteristic at a disadvantage.

Example

The ward has just stated that *all* registered nurses must take their turn to rotate to night duty. Fiaza has children and her husband already works at night. She will need to leave her job or pay for someone to look after the children overnight.

Discrimination by perception

It is also unlawful to discriminate against someone because you *think* they have a protected characteristic, even if they do not. This is called discrimination by perception.

Example

A member of staff refuses to supervise student Alex because they believe that they are transexual.

Associative discrimination

Associative discrimination occurs when someone is discriminated against because they have an association with someone with a protected characteristic.

Example

Lucy has just qualified and is applying for her first job. However, for every job for which she applies, she is not shortlisted. Lucy suspects this is because she has a disabled daughter who has recurring health problems.

Unconscious bias

Healthcare professionals would not wish to be considered discriminatory but, since they are human, they are prone to the same unconscious biases as everyone else (Bucknor-Ferron and Zagaja 2016). Unconscious bias, also known as implicit bias, can be defined as stereotypical beliefs influencing our decisions and behaviours. Unconscious bias is unintentional, often despite a person's best intentions (Bucknor-Ferron and Zagaja 2016). Our unconscious mind is shaped while young, by our cultural background, environment and personal experiences, and we use this information to make quick decisions about everything around us. Everyone will have unconscious preferences for some of the groups discussed within the protected characteristics. This prejudice can also include deep-seated views on social status, education and the way people talk to name but a few examples. Making decisions about care based on these prejudices can be devastating for patients. If unrecognised and unchallenged, such biases have the potential to deepen healthcare disparity.

If unconscious bias is hard to recognise, how can it be challenged? According to Veesart and Barron (2020), the first step is to acknowledge that you have unconscious biases. You can reflect on this yourself or with another person or group, but make sure you are in a safe space and comfortable before starting this conversation. Next, you need to commit to changing your biases actively. Challenge yourself to recognise the biased language used in clinical practice. Make a conscious decision not to perpetuate stereotypes, such as calling the mature and experienced nurses '*old nurses*' and refrain from engaging in conversations about '*troublesome*' patients. Instead, develop empathy with patients and their situation. Importantly, educate yourself. Read about unconscious bias and attend any sessions offered by your education provider or within your clinical area.

Over to you

Can you surface your unconscious biases?

In a calm, relaxed environment, reflect on any unconscious biases you might have. Veesart and Barron (2020) suggest that mindfulness is helpful in allowing you to empty your mind of distraction and leaving space to concentrate on your reflection.

In this section, we have explored the Equality Act (2010), the protected characteristics and different forms of discrimination, conscious and unconscious. In the next section, we present the role that organisations play in supporting patients and staff.

Institutional position on equality, diversity and inclusion

The Equality Act 2010 protects people from discrimination in the workplace and in wider society. Healthcare organisations and education institutions involved in educating nurses are required to adhere to these legal requirements. Below are examples of organisations that you may be familiar with. We outline their responsibilities in relation to EDI.

The Nursing and Midwifery Council

Many healthcare professions hold registration with a professional body who define the standards expected of their registrants. As the regulatory body for nursing and midwifery, the NMC Code of Professional Conduct (NMC 2018) controls initial access to the profession through regulating and monitoring nurse education programmes, and through ensuring registered nurses are fit for practise through continuing professional developments and revalidation. EDI is embedded in the Code as specific items, as seen here.

> ### Green flag
>
> **Item 1.5** Respect and uphold peoples' human rights.
>
> **Item 20.2** To act with honesty and integrity at all times, treating people fairly and without discrimination, bullying or harassment.
>
> **Item 20.7** To 'Make sure you do not express your personal beliefs (including political, religious or moral beliefs) to people in an inappropriate way'.
>
> NMC Code of Professional Conduct (2018)

The NMC Code requires nurses to uphold the values of equality diversity and inclusion. Item 1 states that nurses must 'treat people as individuals and uphold their dignity'. Item 1.5 says that to do this the nurse must 'respect and uphold people's human rights'. Item 20 asks nurses to: 'uphold the reputation of their profession at all times'. This includes, in item 20.2 to: 'act with honesty and integrity at all times, treating people fairly and without discrimination, bullying, or harassment' and in item 20.7 to: 'make sure you do not express your personal beliefs (including political, religious or moral beliefs) to people in an inappropriate way' (NMC 2018). Persistent breaches of the Code with regard to EDI can be reported to the NMC and may result in sanctions, including being removed from the list of registered nurses.

> ### Complete this activity now
>
> Access the NMC Code: www.nmc.org.uk/globalassets/sitedocuments/nmc-publications/nmc-code.pdf. Work through the Code and identify any areas that you consider relate to EDI. Share your findings with your practice supervisor when you are next on placement.

The Royal College of Nursing The Royal College of Nursing (RCN) represents nurses as both a professional and educational body and as a trade union. The RCN commits to equality for all, diversity in the workplace, inclusive culture, upholding human rights, ensuring access to learning and development, and reporting and monitoring complaints and breaches (RCN 2022). There are other trade unions supporting healthcare workers, and they too have their own guidance in accordance with the Equality Act (2010).

Write here

Investigate what support a professional body/trade union (i.e. RCN, UNISON, UNITE) might offer a student nurse who is seeking support related to a disability.

The National Health Service

The NHS has a statutory duty to ensure EDI in everything it does. NHS trusts and other healthcare providers have their own EDI codes of conduct. These codes include information on the standards of behaviour expected of employees, information on how to report breaches, and information on disciplinary procedures following breaches. Some organisations also have formal networks or employee committees for some groups such as ethnic minorities, disability and gender inclusion. Such networks monitor EDI issues, provide information and liaise with employers and staff.

Charitable organisations

Many 'not for profit' and charitable organisations represent the interests of people with a wide range of EDI issues. For example, disability charities are concerned with support, research and treatment; many also act to campaign for equality on behalf of the group they represent. Age UK is a large charity supporting the rights and needs of older people. There are groups that support LGBGTQ+ interests, such as Stonewall. Charities can sometimes be overlooked, but many are extremely active and run successful campaigns in support of EDI issues specific to healthcare.

Higher education organisations

The Council of Deans

As a student in higher education, you will benefit from EDI commitment from both your clinical practice provider and your education establishment. The Council of Deans of Health aims to influence policy and advance healthcare education specifically by sharing and promoting equitable practices.

Advance HE

Advance HE is a charity that works with higher education institutions to improve education for staff, students and society. Under the Equality Act 2010, higher education institutions are required to make reasonable adjustments to students' study environment to ensure equity in the way students learn and are assessed. Advance HE presents examples of reasonable adjustments for students studying nursing. For example, in agreement between the student, the institution and/or the placement provider, students may be supported with additional time for assessments, use additional information technology (IT) such as devices to record handovers, amplified stethoscopes and iPads, and flexible placement hours.

Go online
You might find this link helpful:

Competence standards and reasonable adjustments: nursing – https://
www.advance-he.ac.uk/guidance/equality-diversity-and-inclusion/
student-recruitment-retention-and-attainment/inclusive-learning-and-
teaching/competence-standards-nursing.

Try this on placement

If you need additional support while you are on placement in relation to a protected characteristic, who would you contact to offer you support and why?

So far, we have looked at the legal requirements of organisations in supporting EDI for patients and staff. In the next section, we focus on care for patients that is culturally sensitive to their needs.

Culturally sensitive care

Providing culturally sensitive care

EDI effects many aspects of healthcare provision. Most commonly you might hear this referred to as care that takes a patient's culture into consideration (Congress 2005). The RCN (2022) has a set of eight principles that encompass the provision of nursing care. Two of these principles discuss the importance of nurses providing care that considers the specific needs and wishes of the person or family and providing personalised care ensuring dignity and respect. Provision of care that is respectful, holistic and takes into account what is important to the patient is embedded in policy and standards throughout the UK. Examples can be seen in the NMC Code of Conduct for Nurses, Midwives and Nursing Associates (NMC 2018), NHS training and policy (NHS England 2022), in private healthcare (CQC 2017) and in National Institute for Health and Care Excellence (NICE) guidelines (NICE 2021). All these organisations discuss the importance of providing individualised, holistic and respectful care based on cultural values and beliefs important to a patient and their family.

Traditional definitions of culture have stemmed from considerations of ethnicity and race; however, when regarded as a worldview or having beliefs, values and practices, the concept of culture can be related to many social groups. All humans have culture that is developed through living and interacting with those around them (Stein-Parbury 2021, p. 82). However, culture is often seen, or thought of, as something outside of what is considered normal for you and your family or social group; something that belongs to 'others'.

What is culturally sensitive care?

Within nursing and healthcare, terms such as 'culturally competent care', 'culturally sensitive care', 'culturally congruent care' and 'culturally appropriate care' are used interchangeably but all have an underlying meaning of care provision that takes into account the beliefs, values and practices that are important to the family or person being cared for. This may mean that the person in your care may have values, beliefs and practices different from your own (Stein-Parbury 2021, p. 81). Practically, culture may be represented in language, art, faith or religion, or traditions for life events, raising children, music, clothing and perspectives on medicine, to name but a few.

For patients, clients and their families, being cared for by nurses who understand their culture and what is important to them can reduced stress and increase care satisfaction (Ross et al. 2018; Mutair et al. 2019). In contrast, not actively acknowledging the culture of patients and the local population can lead to health inequalities (Stein-Parbury 2021, p. 82), inaccurate assessment (Givler et al. 2022) or even poor care. For example, if you ask a patient about their pain, you might expect that they are going to give you a sincere answer, but cultural differences can make this complicated. The patient might believe their pain is a test of their faith or something to be endured as part of healing. You might have been taught to look for nonverbal signs of pain such a facial grimace or crying, but this might not be culturally appropriate for some patients (Givler et al. 2022). Understanding these differences will help you assess a person's pain – the first step in effective pain management.

As a nursing student, you might be studying somewhere where you are part of the dominant culture, where the people you are working with and caring for are from a similar background to you. As a new healthcare professional, it would be normal to have a narrow perception of what constitutes culture (Claeys et al. 2021). As part of your professional development, it can be helpful to reflect on your own culture and to consider how this has informed your view of the world.

Over to you: Reflect on your own cultural beliefs and practices

- How has your background informed what is important to you?
- What would be the values and beliefs that would be important to you if you were in hospital?
- Would this change if the care was in your home?

What does culturally sensitive care look like in practice?

Before thinking about the practical implications of culturally sensitive care, it is important to be aware that identifying with a specific culture will mean different things for different people. This chapter is a starting point for your development as a practitioner. In practice, the starting point should always be a conversation with the patient and/or their family. Having an awareness of what patients and their families might ask for or might value can aid care planning and provision.

Go online

Explore what the Care Quality Commission says regarding culturally sensitive care: examples of what providing culturally sensitive care means in practice: www.cqc.org.uk/guidance-providers/adult-social-care/culturally-appropriate-care appropriatecare

Table 4.1 provides examples of some questions you might find helpful to consider when caring for all patients. These suggested questions are just a starting point and not an exhaustive list of possibilities.

Over to you

What other questions would you add?

TABLE 4.1

How to: some questions to ask patients and families.

Area of care	Potential questions
General admission or when meeting the person for the first time	Is there anything that is important to you that I/we can support you with during your care? Will anyone be visiting during your stay? How can I/we support your communication?
Food and drink	Do you have any dietary restrictions? Do you need your meals at a specific time? Are there likely to be any changes to your diet while I/we are caring for you?

(Continued)

TABLE **4.1**

(Continued)

Area of care	Potential questions
Personal care	How would you like me/us to support your personal care? How would you like me/us to care for and style your hair? Do you have any skincare regimens that are important to you? Do you have any preferences with regards to the staff supporting you with your personal care?
Spirituality and faith	Is there anything I/we can do to support your spirituality while I/we are caring for you? Are there any specific times of day you need me/us to be aware of? Do you need a specific place for prayers? Are there any upcoming dates I/we need to be aware of?
Medication	Are you aware of any medications that would not be acceptable to you? Do you observe any periods of fasting? Are there any specific times of day that would be difficult to take medication or that you would like to avoid?

When patient's values are in conflict with your own

Acknowledging and being respectful of a person's worldview or culture when it is different from our own can be challenging. As professionals, we have a duty to be nonjudgemental and not to inappropriately express our views and opinions to those in our care (NMC 2021). For example, you might be an atheist who is providing palliative care for a patient and family who are practising Catholics (or vice versa). Espousing your views might cause distress resulting in them feeling unsupported.

There might be circumstances where you do not feel able to undertake care for someone based on your own beliefs. The first course of action would be to discuss this with your practice assessor/practice supervisor in placement and your personal tutor/academic assessor. In certain circumstances, there are legal grounds for your objecting to providing care based on your beliefs (NMC 2021).

What if I see something I do not think is respectful of a patient's culture?

Care that is culturally sensitive can be complex and there can be challenges to care delivery in practice. Some barriers reported in research concern staff knowledge and awareness, staff experience and attitude, as well as policies and procedures (Phillips et al. 2019; van Herwaarden et al. 2020). Although not widely cited in the literature, time constraints are likely to be another challenge for culturally sensitive care initially, as a thorough discussion about cultural needs with a patient and their family will take longer than an assessment that does not consider this fact.

Examples such as failure to provide appropriate food, not supporting external visitors or having overly rigid routines, and thus not acknowledging or supporting a patient or client's culture, could be categorised as institutional abuse (Social Care Institute of Excellence 2015). Institutional abuse is a category considered under safeguarding laws. In healthcare, safeguarding both adults and children is everyone's responsibility (RCN 2018) and if a colleague or professional is deliberately disregarding someone's culture, and you think there might be a safeguarding concern, you should look at the organisation or trusts safeguarding policy. You can also talk to your education provider, practice assessor/practice supervisor in placement and your personal tutor/academic assessor or programme leader for support. You might also find the organisation's Raising a Concern policy helpful, or the NMC whistleblowing guidelines (NMC 2022).

Complete this activity now

Go online and access this site: Raising a whistleblowing concern (https://protect-advice.org.uk/raising-a-concern).

Make notes about what you would do if you have seen something that concerns you at work but you are not sure how or whether you should whistleblow.

How to advocate for your own equality, diversity and inclusion requirements

The NMC (2020) EDI strategic framework priorities serve to support patients and clients by challenging discrimination, reducing health inequalities, improving the evidence-base for the services we provide and improving nurses' knowledge in providing culturally competent care. The strategy also focuses on the EDI needs of healthcare staff and students by ensuring their wellbeing through an inclusive workplace culture. Importantly, the NMC (2019) guidance on health and character makes it clear that all nurses (registered or a student) have a responsibility to self-declare that they are in 'good health' and capable of safe and effective practice, with or without reasonable adjustments made by the education establishment or practice areas. As a student, you are required to tell your education institution about any health conditions or disabilities that might affect your ability to meet the requirements to study on a nursing or midwifery programme.

A supervisor's notes

Ailsa (a first-year mental health nursing student) was allocated to our general practice for a six-week placement. I first met her when she came for an informal visit in preparation for the placement. I was to be her practice supervisor. When Alisa arrived after the second day, we sat down to undertake the first interview for the placement identifying Ailsa's learning needs and any other needs she may have. During our discussion, Ailsa revealed that she had type 1 diabetes. We sat down and made a tailored plan to ensure that Ailsa felt supported and would be able to complete her placement successfully. We would, if needed, put in place reasonable adjustments, such a regular food-time breaks. This was a great experience for all of us; we all learned from having a student who had needs that she made us aware of. She taught so much about diabetes from her own perspective. It is kind of like sitting with a patient in surgery and asking them 'how can we best help you', 'what can we do for you'. I am pleased to say her placement with us was a huge success.

Jorge, practice nurse

Just as nurses advocate for patients, they also need to advocate for their own EDI needs. Self-advocacy is about speaking up for yourself and making your own choices. Student nurses are encouraged to be proactive in their learning journey and to get the best out of their learning environments (higher education setting, or in clinical practice; Downer et al. 2022). If you have a disability or feel disadvantaged or otherwise adversely affected due to any protected characteristic(s), how do you advocate for *your* needs? McCulloch and Marks (2016) suggest that, where possible, you should ensure that those involved in your nurse education programme are aware of your situation as soon as possible. This enables support to be put in place quickly. Communicating your needs effectively and being confident is key to self-advocacy, according to Downer et al. (2022).

Managing effective self-advocacy

To illustrate how self-advocacy might be achieved, below are real examples from students who ensured their needs were supported while studying and working in clinical areas. All the students below have protected characteristics according to the Equality Act 2010. The students' names have been changed to protect anonymity.

Hear it from the students

- Gina was pregnant during year one of her adult nursing course. She was worried about how she would juggle studying, placement and being a mum to two small children. She felt unwell at the start of her pregnancy and had to take time off. This was affecting a pending exam. She did not know if she would be able to continue on the course.
- Alison, a second year adult nurse, has a disability. Alison's main concern was about her levels of tiredness and how she might manage her commute daily to her practice placement. She was also worried about how she would cope with a 12-hour shift as she had never been on her feet for that long before.
- Zainab is a second year children's nurse. Her Muslim faith is very important to her and she upholds religious practices in her day-to-day life. She dresses modestly but recognises that there are some challenges to this when practising as a nurse. In Islam, a Muslim woman should cover all parts of her body in the presence of non-mahram people (people who are not family). Zainab wanted to cover her arms but, for infection control reasons, healthcare staff must have their arms exposed below the elbow.

Be self-aware

The better you understand your needs, the more effective you can be in obtaining help and support for them. Be clear about what you need and communicate it effectively. Be prepared to describe your disability or needs relating to your protected characteristic(s).

All the students spoke to their personal tutor at university in the first instance. In all cases, this communication initiated the process of support.

Hear it from the student

The first person I told was my personal tutor, who did a risk assessment to make sure I was safe while at university. I then had a useful conversation with the student welfare team, who helped me decide the best time to return to university once the baby was born. I also found out what support was available with regard to my upcoming exam (additional tutorials and extenuating circumstances).

Gina, adult nurse year 2

Be assertive and know your rights

Know your rights and be prepared to take responsibility for meeting some of your needs. You may need to find creative solutions when none are available. Alison was already aware of her rights with regard to her disability. She was proactive in ensuring support was in place before she started on her nursing course. Zainab investigated the trust's uniform policy before going on her first placement.

Hear it from the student

I had been at this university before, so I already had a disability statement in place. Before I started the nursing course, I decided to get this updated as my last degree did not have placements. The disability support team at university were really good and they talked to the placement office on my behalf to make sure I went to a local placement.

Alison, adult nurse year 2

> When we are not providing patient care, I believe that students like myself can have the responsibility to choose to cover their arms when walking around the hospital. It is written in the trust's uniform policy about the use of sleeves; however, I was surprised to find out that they are not readily available in clinical areas. Better still would be for us to be able to request uniforms with three-quarter sleeves when we start the course.
>
> Zainab, children's nurse year 2

Be self-confident

Be confident when sharing your situation with others. Make sure you are listened to, and if you are not satisfied with the help on offer, be prepared to say so. While it is advised to discuss needs at the start of each placement, Alison feels confident in sharing information when *she* feels ready to do so. Zainab decided to speak out and about not being able to find disposable sleeves. However, she knows she needs to be confident to be able to make this request at new placements.

Hear it from the student

Personally, I have made the decision not to tell placement staff as soon as I arrive. This just suits me. I prefer to chat about it more informally with staff if a situation arises of if they ask. This works best for me.

Alison, adult nurse year 2

> I spoke with my personal tutor about where I might be able to find some disposable sleeves. My tutor and I talked to the placement practice facilitators and the ward manager. Sleeves were arranged for me on this placement. However, not all trusts have them in their uniform policy. It looks like I may have to go through this if I change trust. I fully understand that patient safety is to be my first priority but this can be done while practising my faith.
>
> Zainab, children's nurse year 2

Accept the help available

Do not feel afraid to ask for help or to accept what is offered to you. Gemma found that she had lots of support from the whole ward team.

Hear it from the student

On the first day of my new placement, the ward manager and I completed a risk assessment together. She was really supportive and advised me on what activities I could do and what I should avoid. All the ward staff kept telling me to 'sit down'. They were so supportive. I was allowed to decide on my own break times and could take snack breaks when I needed.

I left the course at the end of year one. Ruby was born in December. I took a year away from university and returned at the start of year 2.

Gina, adult nurse year 2

Go online

Explore what the NMC says about health and character: *Guidance on Health and Character* (NMC 2019): www.nmc.org.uk/globalassets/ sitedocuments/nmc-publications/guidance-on-health-and-character

Summary

In this chapter, we have illustrated the importance of understanding protected characteristics as defined by the Equality Act 2010 and have highlighted how discriminatory behaviour might negatively impact on the health and wellbeing of patients, families, healthcare providers and wider society. Organisations are legally required to ensure equity within healthcare and in your education journey as a student nurse. Nurses need to be aware of cultural differences when providing care. They need to be compassionate, culturally informed and curious about individuals. Inability to do this can lead to poor satisfaction with healthcare provision and health inequalities. Nurses also need to be aware of their own health needs and to ensure that they are in good health when caring for others. Meeting your own EDI needs requires assertiveness and effective communication skills.

Acknowledgements

With thanks to the students who gave their time to tell us their stories.

References

Amnesty International (2023), Discrimination. https://www.amnesty.org/en/what-we-do/discrimination (accessed 15 March 2023).

Bachmann, C.L. and Gooch, B. (2018). *LGBT in Britain: Trans Report.* London: Stonewall.

Bucknor-Ferron, P. and Zagaja, L. (2016). Five strategies to combat unconscious bias. *Nursing* 46 (11): 61–62. https://doi.org/10.1097/01.NURSE.0000490226.81218.6c.

Care Quality Commission (2017). Inspection Report for HCA Healthcare at University College Hospital. https://api.cqc.org.uk/public/v1/reports/182d6a51-1fd0-40fd-b26b-533346b27fa9?20210119011407 (accessed 25 November 2022).

Care Quality Commission (2022). Culturally appropriate care. www.cqc.org.uk/guidance-providers/adult-social-care/culturally-appropriate-care   appropriatecare (accessed 11 June 2022).

Claeys, A., Berdai-Chaouni, S., Tricas-Sauras, S., and De Donder, L. (2021). Culturally sensitive care: definitions, perceptions, and practices of health care professionals. *Journal of Transcultural Nursing* 32 (5): 484–492.

Congress, E.P. (2005). Cultural and ethical issues in working with culturally diverse patients and their families: the use of the culturagram to promote cultural competent practice in health care settings. *Social Work in Health Care* 39 (4): 249–262.

Downer, M., Walpuri, J., Rouid, G. et al. (2022). *Self-Advocacy: An Important Skill for Students on Clinical Placement.* Wellington, New Zealand: Kaitiaki Nursing.

Givler, A., Bhatt, H., and Maani-Fogelman, P.A. (2022). The Importance Of Cultural Competence in Pain and Palliative Care. Treasure Island (FL): StatPearls Publishing. www.ncbi.nlm.nih.gov/books/NBK493154 (accessed 27 November 2022).

McCulloch, K. and Marks, D. (2016). *Challenges and Strategies of Nursing Students with Disabilities*, 66–67. New Hampshire Nurse.

Mutair, A.A., Ammary, M.A., Brooks, L.A., and Bloomer, M.J. (2019). Supporting Muslim families before and after a death in neonatal and paediatric intensive care units. *Nursing and Critical Care* 24: 192–200.

National Institute for Health and Care Excellence (2021). Patient experience in adult NHS services: improving the experience of care for people using adult NHS services. www.nice.org.uk/guidance/cg138/chapter/1-guidance (accessed 27 November 2022).

NHS England (2022). Equality objectives and information as at 30 March 2021. https://www.england.nhs.uk/publication/equality-objectives-and-information-as-at-30-march-2021 (accessed on: 16 November 2022).

Nursing and Midwifery Council (2018). The Code: Professional standards of practice and behaviour for nurses, midwives and nursing associates. www.nmc.org.uk/standards/code/read-the-code-online (accessed 27 November 2022).

Nursing and Midwifery Council (2019). Guidance on Health and Character. www.nmc.org.uk/globalassets/sitedocuments/nmc-publications/guidance-on-health-and-character (accessed 15 March 2023).

Nursing and Midwifery Council (2020). NMC Strategy 2020–2025. www.nmc.org.uk/about-us/our-role/our-strategy (accessed 15 March 2023).

Nursing and Midwifery Council (2021). Conscientious objection by nurses and midwives. www.nmc.org.uk/standards/code/conscientious-objection-by-nurses-and-midwives (accessed 28 November 2022).

Nursing and Midwifery Council (2022). Whistleblowing to the NMC. www.nmc.org.uk/standards/guidance/raising-concerns-guidance-for-nurses-and-midwives/whistleblowing/#:~:text=Whistleblowing%20is%20when%20a%20worker,as%20a%20'prescribed%20person (accessed 28 November 2022).

Phillips, S., Villalobos, A.V.K., Crawbuck, G.S.N., and Pratt-Chapman, M.L. (2019). In their own words: patient navigator roles in culturally sensitive cancer care. *Supportive Care in Cancer* 27: 1655–1662.

Public Health England (2018). Local action on health inequalities: Understanding and reducing ethnic in equalities in health. https://assets.publishing.service.gov.uk/government/uploads/system/uploads/attachment_data/file/730917/local_action_on_health_inequalities.pdf (accessed 15 March 2023).

Ross, L., McSherry, W., Giste, T. et al. (2018). Nursing and midwifery students' perceptions of spirituality, spiritual care, and spiritual care competency: a prospective, longitudinal, correlational European study. *Nurse Education Today* 67: 64–71.

Royal College of Nursing (2018). Adult Safeguarding: Roles and Competencies for Health Care Staff. www.rcn.org.uk/Professional-Development/publications/adult-safeguarding-roles--and-competencies-for-health-care-staff-uk-pub-007-069 (accessed 28 November 2022).

Royal College of Nursing (2021). RCN Group. Equality, Diversity and Inclusion Statement Diversity and Inclusion. www.rcn.org.uk/About-us/Diversity-and-inclusion (accessed 15 March 2023).

Royal College of Nursing (2022). Principles of Nursing Practice. www.rcn.org.uk/Professional-Development/publications/pub-003864 (accessed 11 June 2022).

Social Care Institute of Excellence (2015). Types and Indicators of Abuse. www.scie.org.uk/safeguarding/adults/introduction/types-and-indicators-of-abuse#discriminatory (accessed 28 November 2022).

Stein-Parbury, J. (2021). *Patient and Person: Interpersonal Skills in Nursing*, 7e. Amsterdam: Elsevier.

Veesart, A. and Barron, A. (2020). Unconscious bias: is it impacting your nursing care? *Nursing Made Easy* 18: 47–49.

van Herwaarden, A., Rommes, E.W., and Peters-Scheffer, N.C. (2020). Providers' perspectives on factors complicating the culturally sensitive care of individuals with intellectual disabilities. *Research in Developmental Disabilities* 96: 103543.

Further Reading

E-Learning for Health (n.d.). Available at: *Home - elearning for healthcare (e*-http://lfh.org. uk), (Accessed on: 20/11/2022)

Guterres, A. (2019). *United Nations Strategy and Plan of Action on Hate Speech*. Geneva: United Nations.

CHAPTER 5

Learning in practice

Lucy Tyler and Paulette Ragan

AIM

This chapter intends to support the reader in providing an insight in what to expect from clinical placement and how to maximise learning and development while in clinical practice placements.

LEARNING OUTCOMES

Having read this chapter, the reader will:

1. Understand how learning in practice differs from learning in the classroom or online.
2. Be able to discuss where learning might take place.
3. Be able to describe the types of learning opportunity that may present themselves.
4. Be able to describe ways of teaching and facilitation of learning-simulation/hybrid learning.
5. Have an understanding of simulation-based learning within clinical practice.

Succeeding on your Nursing Placement: Supervision, Learning and Assessment for Nursing Students, First Edition. Edited by Ian Peate.
© 2024 John Wiley & Sons Ltd. Published 2024 by John Wiley & Sons Ltd.

Introduction

The history of learning in practice can be traced back to the very inception of modern nursing. Those with an enthusiasm for history will be aware that Florence Nightingale, often described as the mother of modern nursing practice, proved the worth of nursing during the Crimean war in the 1860s. Before this, the sick and dying were cared for by servants or family members. These individuals were untrained, although some would have gained valuable experience from caring for multiple patients and would have had a good knowledge of folk medicine and how to induce feelings of comfort and were able to show compassion.

The ruling classes faired better than their less affluent counterparts, and for those resident sick patients in the poor houses of the time, good luck alone would bring you a kind and gentle individual to tend to you in your hour of need. However, for the most part, the caring community was made up of untrained individuals, mostly female and, as Florence Nightingale described them, 'slatterns, and drunks'.

Following the Crimean war, all of this changed. Florence Nightingale set up a school of nursing at St Thomas's Hospital, located in the London Borough of Lambeth. The actual practice of training nurses at the time involved cleaning the ward environment, washing bedding, personal care, moving and handling, administration of medication, wound care and dressing changes. This is not entirely dissimilar to what and how learner nurses are taught today; in this chapter, we expand on where some changes may have taken place in line with learning and teaching theory.

In the clinical context, during training in the early 1990s skills were taught through a process of learning in practice; minimal time throughout the three-year programme was spent in the classroom. Students took part in a widely experiential learning process that offered the valuable opportunity to learn by doing alongside a more experienced nurse. This apprenticeship-style route to registration offered very different types of learning, including occupational socialisation into the ward environment and into the culture of nursing itself. Opportunities for learning presented themselves constantly; passive learning in the clinical environment was commonplace but undocumented. Consistently present were the multidisciplinary team, allocated mentors of more senior and experienced nurses, and there was huge potential for drawing on non-technical clinical skills such as negotiation with patients, picking up clinical terminology and gaining a depth of understanding. Much of this learning activity takes place in twenty-first century nurse education but over a shorter timescale; clinical placements are shorter with a more academic focus.

With this historical context in mind, this chapter reviews learning in practice as the dominant form of education for UK nurses and how this now manifests as we enter an era of ever-evolving technology in the healthcare sector as well as in educational institutions.

Timespans of nurse education may vary, but the Nursing and Midwifery Council (NMC) requires the learner to cover a minimum of 2300 hours of clinical practice before registration. This ensures that learners are prepared for joining the workforce with the required knowledge, skills and ability to safely and professionally fulfil their roles. In addition, this learning is assessed carefully using several different and ever evolving methods. Reading, writing and experiential learning remain the mainstay of education. Over more recent years, there has been an introduction of alternative methods such as clinical simulation, virtual reality and other forms of synthesis. Simulation (or 'sim') laboratories account for significant proportions of training budgets and are built into almost every learning and healthcare institution.

Summary

This section has provided an historical overview, acknowledging that we are entering an era of ever-evolving technology in the healthcare sector and also in educational institutions.

How learning in practice differs from learning in the classroom or online

The practice environment offers a variety of opportunities for pre-registration and post registration students for learning clinical and non-clinical skills by observing and participating in practice-based activities. Nurses post registration learn how to facilitate the learning of others in the clinical environment through peer feedback, a requirement of the NMC (2019).

Auditing placement by the universities proves the suitability of the placement. The approved education institution or higher education institution, with its practice learning partners, must ensure that all such placements have proper oversight and governance. This can be done in a few different ways, such as through documentation, audits and visits. (NMC 2019).

At first, the concept of the difference of learning in practice, as opposed to working online or in the classroom, seems obvious. Students are involved in 'learning by doing'; they absorb methods of 'doing' by observing more experienced students and staff in their work activities and therefore perpetuate cultures of the practice they have seen carried out within the specialism and across wider clinical learning environments. Students will experience a hands-on experience, where they will be required to take part in the layers of activity that make up an interaction between nurse and patient, as well as governing communication with the multidisciplinary team (MDT) and ensuring the patients' needs are met.

Hughes and Quinn (2013) suggest that students will pick up clinical and non-clinical skills; the practice-based placement is a crucial factor in the absorption of these skills over the period of the educational period. However, there may be less obvious areas of learning taking place in the practice environment that are also essential and differ from the more structured learning environment.

Practice settings vary a great deal in the UK for student nurses and all offer their own unique sets of culture, styles and formats for learning. Following the COVID-19 pandemic, clinical placement has become increasingly pressurised due to several factors: placements are further stretched and therefore they are few and far between. This has led to innovative and creative ideas being generated by educational staff around how to bridge the gap between practice and theory.

Example

An interesting and alternative example of learning through observation is presented in the training of the Japanese raw fish or sushi chefs. Training to become a sushi chef takes around 10 years. Trainees are prohibited from interacting with the fish in any way for the first two years of training; they simply remain in the sushi kitchen environment to observe the work of the senior qualified chefs closely. After two years, they may be allowed to carry out the preparation of the raw fish.

Activity

- Can you name a time recently when you have been working in placement and have observed a more senior nurse or student carrying out a skill or action?
- How many times did you feel you needed to observe that skill before you could carry it out yourself with supervision? What did this depend on?
- Did you notice how each individual practitioner performed the skill in a slightly or widely different way? What did this tell you about developing your own style?
- How does this effect the principles of the skill?

We are reminded by Fernandez (1997) that direct observation is one of the best ways to assess how a person practices. However, in healthcare there are many occasions when being observed with clients is neither practical nor ethical, yet clinical expertise is built upon these experiences, critical incidents and turning points in a career. Despite the embedded and historical traditions attached to nurse education in the UK, several different models have begun to emerge as a response to changes taking place in the healthcare system as detailed above.

Student nurses learning in the clinical environment is described by Hill et al. (2020) as the method by which knowledge, skills and abilities are safely and effectively learnt. The Royal College of Nursing (RCN) commissioned the Willis Report in 2012, which found that learning placements could be variable in quality but acknowledged that practice placements were central to creating a compassionate and competent workforce.

The Willis Report

The Willis Report (2012) undertook an assessment of the standards of care in nursing and healthcare. The commission looked at how the care needs of service users were changing and how nurse education needed to review preparation for the future and how future proofing the profession was essential.

One year later, the Francis Report (2013) was published as a result of a government-commissioned investigation into the failings of the Mid Staffordshire NHS Trust to care adequately for service users. The Francis Report brought about significant cultural change within the NHS, and there was a recognition that the issues that effected the trust could have happened at any other trust or care setting nationally. Together with several other reports of around the same time, namely the Keogh (2013), Bubb (2014) and Berwick (2013) Reports, Health Education England published *'Raising the Bar' Shape of Caring: A Review of the Future Education and Training of Registered Nurses and Care Assistants* (Willis 2015).

As a direct result of the Francis Report and others around the same time, the NMC initially introduced a number of changes for nurse education for post registration practitioners, and it was recognised that education for pre-registration nurses was in need of review. In 2018, a new standards framework for nursing was introduced, although in some clinical areas it was postponed due to the increased pressures caused by the COVID-19 global pandemic. The new standards are set out in three parts and focus on the changes needed to futureproof the profession.

Collaborative learning in practice

The collaborative learning in practice (CLIP) model first emerged in 2014 from the Netherlands. The educational style acknowledges the need to support the student but uses a less pedagogical approach and employs coaching to achieve this support. Students are placed in a more responsible position and guided to a balanced decision through assistance from the coach. This method of education has become increasingly popular due to a recent reduction in clinical placements, and is seen as a method of assisting students to develop their professionalism through peer support. Faithfull-Byrne et al. (2017) suggest that using methods of coaching to support the philosophical elements of learning has presented an alternative approach to clinical learning.

Student support becomes a team approach, intended to facilitate growth and development towards registrant practice, with collaboration between nurses who supervise and coach students and greater collaboration between students because there are more students in placement areas. This approach is particularly useful for third-year students, who can lead small teams for care management, and those teams ought to include more junior students, as well as unqualified nursing staff and other learners (Williamson et al. 2020). This has been discussed as improving students' learning and satisfaction with placement (Health Education England 2017, Huggins 2016).

CLIP requires planning, preparation and project management as it requires a cultural change in supporting and assessing learning, delivering care and perpetuating best practice. The GROW model ('goal, reality, options/obstacles, and will/way forward'; Whitmore 2017), used by supervisors and for peer-to-peer coaching by students, underpins learning requiring reflection and reflexivity, which is already embedded into the ethos of nursing and midwifery.

Where learning might take place

Health Education England reported that in 2020, nurse training places in universities had increased by 25.9% from the previous year. In consideration of this fact, the requirement for more diverse learning environments has arisen and this has instigated a wider approach to clinical placement. Clinical placements might now be located in a wide variety of diverse settings. The thinking is that where there is a human health need there is a clinical placement. This opens up a very wide gamut of placement opportunities, including prisons, detention centres, care and nursing homes, localised drug and alcohol projects, general practice and research facilities, as well as spending time with those in higher management positions, such as chief executives of hospital trusts and private sector providers.

The NMC (2019) states that clinical learning takes place through learning opportunities. These opportunities are divided into:

- *Group learning* – students spend time learning as a group, which creates opportunities to learn together as well as identifying the emergent strengths of members of the group (i.e. leaders, public speakers, ideas person, researchers).
- *One-to-one learning* – learning with one other person – is preferred by some students, depending on their learning style and preference.
- *Peer-to-peer learning* might take place more often in placement settings, where other students and newly qualified nurses are present.
- *Direct patient care*, as the name suggests, will take place in clinical settings.

Box 5.1 describes a case study to encourage you to learn more about learning in practice.

Box 5.1 | Passive learning in practice

Jesse is a student nurse starting out in trauma and orthopaedics at the very beginning of the second year of nurse education. His day starts with the handover, with registered members of staff and two fellow students, who are in their first and third years of nurse education.

During the handover, Jesse observes the use of the term 'NOF' on the whiteboard on the wall in the room. He requests the meaning of the abbreviation at this point and is informed that this is a shortening for neck of femur. The nurse in charge of the shift informs the staff that the use of the abbreviation has its place but that this is poor practice and prevents more junior staff and students from gaining required knowledge.

Later in the shift, Jesse is asked to accompany a patient and a member of staff to the operating theatre. Before leaving the ward, the staff member introduces Jesse to a checklist for ensuring that the correct patient is being taken for their operation and begins to ask the patient questions. During this time, he observes the body language of the patient, and he appears tense. While the nurse gathers the required paperwork for theatre, Jesse chats with the patient and learns that he is very nervous about going for surgery.

Jesse returns to the ward and is invited to look through the patient's notes. He can hear the physiotherapist speaking with a junior doctor at the nurse's station. They are discussing a patient who needs to be encouraged to walk with a nurse to the toilet rather than being offered a bed pan or commode.

Complete this activity now

Using the scenario in Box 5.1, reflect on where and how learning may have taken place:

- Record what you think that Jesse may have learnt.
- How is this useful to Jesse in terms of his practice?
- Is all the learning noted here passive learning?
- What other types of learning can you identify?

Types of learning opportunities in practice

While on placement, there are many learning opportunities to enhance your learning and development. As a student, you will work collaboratively with those within the placement area to support and facilitate learning opportunities, as well as seeking learning opportunities as part of your own learning and development. In this section, we discuss several types of learning opportunities available to you while you are in practice.

Everyday learning opportunities

Everyday learning opportunities involve all the learning opportunities available to you within the placement area, such as the everyday tasks and activities within the placement area for you to achieve the proficiencies as outlined in your practice placement assessment document (see Chapter 9); for example, undertaking vital signs, being involved in personal hygiene activities with patients and assisting with feeding or medication administration. Box 5.2 gives some tips for getting the most out of learning in practice and achieving all the required learning outcomes.

Box 5.2 | How to ensure you are getting the most out of learning in practice and achieving all the required learning outcomes

A good tip is to think daily about what you would like to achieve within a shift and to communicate this with your practice supervisor, assessor or any other staff member with whom you are working, preferably at the start, and that you would like feedback. Think about what your learning outcomes are for the day and how you could achieve them and what specifically you would like feedback on.

An example

You might decide that you need to work on your medication administration, especially the procedure, using the rights of medication administration and drug calculations. You could achieve this by observing your practice assessor/supervisor for one medication administration, then you could undertake medication administration under the supervision of your assessor and gaining feedback for future improvements, especially around drug calculations and how you used the rights of medication administration.

Complete this activity now

Complete this activity at the start of your first placement. You may also find it beneficial to complete the activity again at the start of each of your placements.

Think about and list all day-to-day learning activities in which you could be involved while on placement:

Specific learning opportunities

Specific learning opportunities involve certain learning opportunities and experiences that you might get only from a particular practice placement. An example of this is observing a surgical procedure, such a total hip replacement while in an orthopaedic ward or spending a day with the ambulance crew during a placement in the emergency department. Or it might involve a certain examination undertaken specifically within the placement environment; for example, using the Glasgow coma scale assessment on a neurological ward where it is part of their daily practice with this patient group. These types of learning opportunities are valuable to your learning and development due to the insight and knowledge they provide you about the patient's journey and what this could mean as part of the care the patient receives, as well as extending your learning and development in a particular patient group and allowing you the opportunity to learn and develop other essential skills and being supported by experts in that field.

Complete this activity now

Think about your next placement and try to list all the learning opportunities specific to the placement area. In the future, you might want to repeat this activity to compare what you thought the learning opportunities were with what was actually available.

Learning from other health and care professionals

While learning in practice, there are many opportunities for you to gain insight and knowledge from other health and care professionals. As healthcare professionals, we work as a team, so it is essential that you gain an insight and knowledge about what other professionals do. This may also include other nurse specialists who are involved in patient care; for example, an epilepsy nurse specialist will work very closely with the neurologist and nurses on the neurology ward to ensure a safe discharge and continuing care and treatment of a patient who has epilepsy. Another example is that, while on a community placement, you may be working very closely with social workers, specialist medical teams and general practitioners, and the role of the nurse may be coordinating with all these different health and social care teams to ensure patient-centred care and being an advocate for the patient. You can see how essential it is for you to develop an understanding of what other healthcare professionals do to ensure the best possible care for the patient.

Try this on placement

While on your next placement, ensure that you work and learn from other health and care professionals linked to the placement area to find out what their role is, what they do and how they work with the rest of the MDT. Think about how referrals are made and what the role of the nurse is within the MDT.

> ### Green flag
>
> You can record all the different learning opportunities you undertake with any healthcare professional in your placement assessment documents. You can discuss what you learnt, how it will support your future practice, and you can ask the healthcare professional for feedback for you. This is an excellent way of demonstrating how you are developing and enhancing your learning while in practice.

Simulation-based learning opportunities in practice

Simulation-based learning is an excellent way to enhance your learning experience and provides you with opportunities to put into practice knowledge and skills learnt in a safe way. See Chapter 3 of this text for further discussion of simulated based learning.

Most healthcare trusts and settings now have a linked simulation and skills centre supported by trained simulation technicians and clinical staff trained and developing in the use of simulation as an education strategy. Simulation is recognised as an essential strategy in all healthcare education, training and development, and is growing and advancing quickly in all its modalities and fidelities.

In comparison with simulation used in a university setting, within clinical practice you may hear the term 'in situ sim'. This refers to simulations that occur in the clinical environment and focus on scenarios linked to the clinical area. For example, emergency department in situ sims can be used for scenarios that require many different teams who need to be involved in a patient's care, such as maternity emergencies, involving the emergency department team and contacting the maternity and paediatric teams. However, you may have simulation-based learning experiences within the simulation centre that are similar to those you will find within your university.

> ### Try this on placement
>
> While you are on placement, find out if there is a linked simulation and skills centre. Find out what training and development they offer to staff and how you as a student can be involved.

Try this on placement

If being part of a simulation-based activity is an option provided to you, be involved while on placement. If it is not, why not try discussing it with your practice assessor/supervisor or simulation centre staff to see if this is something which could be organised, especially if there is a group of students and a learning need for other staff members identified.

A supervisor's notes

I am often involved in simulation activities. The university where some of our students come from have amazing facilities that really help us to help the students learn in a range of environments. The students get a lot out of these sessions, they really enjoy them, and we can provide them with real-time feedback and feedforward.

Janice, staff nurse

Hear it from the student

Using simulation as a way to learn (for me) is just great – I love it. It really helps me with regards to confidence and helps with my competence. I like the idea of being able to take my time, think about what it is I am doing and, best of all, reflecting on what I have done well and what I could have done better. We always debrief after the sim sessions; people often see things that I have not noticed or even considered.

Manuka, first-year child nurse student

Go online

The following frameworks will provide you with more information about simulation-based education:

• ASPiH (Association of Simulated Practice in Healthcare) sets out a framework of standards that providers of simulation should follow: https://aspih.org.uk/standards-framework-for-sbe

- Health Education England also has a national framework for simulation-based education, which applies to university and clinical practice settings: https://www.hee.nhs.uk/sites/default/files/documents/National%20framework%20for%20simulation%20based%20education.pdf

Opportunistic learning opportunities

Healthcare is forever changing and is at times unpredictable, so opportunities to learn may present themselves to you while you are in placement that you or the placement team had not thought about. An example of this is urinary catherisation. Sometimes you may go lengthy periods of time where this is not a procedure required for a patient, so it is good to seize these types of opportunities when they arrive.

Try this is on placement

How to maximise your opportunistic opportunities

One way to enhance recognition of your opportunities, opportunistic or not often seen clinical skills and/or activities is to introduce yourself and get to know others within your placement area and by sharing skills/activities you would like to be involved in. If they know you would like to part take in a particular skill or experience (e.g. urinary catherisation) then they will make sure to let you know when this procedure/experience is happening for you to either observe, participate or be assessed in.

Learning through facilitating the learning of others

Being able to pass your knowledge on to others is an ideal way to ensure that you have learnt and mastered particular skills. Through facilitating the learning of others, you too are learning, developing and mastering many essential skills required as a nurse, such as communication, teamwork, leadership and facilitating the learning of others. Facilitating the learning of others is part of the NMC Code (2018). As a student, you are in a prime position to know and understand how a fellow student is feeling, knowing what worked for you and supporting them in their development, which will in turn support your development in this area.

Try this on placement

Why not teach a skill or something you have learnt to another student. Reflect on this, what went well? What did not go so well? What was challenging? What would you do differently? What have you learnt from this experience? How did it make you feel?

Structured learning opportunities

Many placement areas, as part of their education policies, will have outlined the many opportunities for you to learn while in their placement area. Some areas may have a specially designed workbook or may have recognised a programme of learning opportunities for you to undertake while there. Make sure that you seek this out and discuss it with your practice assessor, supervisor or education lead so that you know what learning opportunities are available and you maximise your time while in the placement area. This will be linked to your initial and midpoint interviews.

Over to you

Think about your learning needs at the start of a placement and what you need to achieve these learning outcomes. Be specific and focus on one aspect when writing a learning outcome.

An example of a learning outcome

Learning outcome	Requirement to achieve
Be able to undertake a full set of vital signs, document these and report findings to assessors.	Undertake vital signs for a group of patients including documenting results and reporting findings to staff. Have the assessor and other staff observe me and provide feedback on progress.

Learning from service users

Service users (patients, clients) and their friends, family and carers are often experts in their care needs and conditions, illness and symptoms being experienced, providing you with the lived experience from their perspectives. They can provide you with a valuable and unique learning opportunity. As students, you are in a prime position to access service users and their friends, family and carers to ask questions related to them and their healthcare needs and the impact their conditions have on different aspects of their lives. However, we must be mindful of ethics and confidentiality when choosing moments to talk with the service user and what we are asking them. For example, it may not be appropriate to discuss their continuing illness shortly after they have received some upsetting news regarding their treatment and condition. It is important to gain consent that the service user is willing and is able to talk to you and answer your questions. There may be moments when you are performing parts of routine care with the service user, and this may provide a more natural way to engage in conversation and to learn from the service user.

Regarding confidentiality, the NMC Code (2018) specifies that we must respect people's right to privacy and confidentiality; however, we must remember that information may be shared in the interest of patient and others safety.

Try this on placement

Spend some time talking to a service user. Think about what you have learnt from talking to the service user and how it might support your future practice.

Green flag

For every placement, it is a requirement for you to gain feedback from service users. This includes from their family, friends and carers. Ensure that you seek feedback from service users and ask them to be specific in their feedback that they provide you. Maybe ask them to provide you with feedback on a particular aspect of your practice; for example, communicating and providing information on a medication you administered to them.

Summary

In this section, we have discussed the many learning opportunities that are available to you for you to develop and learn whilst in placement.

Green flag

Remember to:

- seek out if the placement area has a planned programme of learning opportunities and or workbook
- think about all the different learning opportunities that may be available to you using the headings provided in this section
- think about your learning outcomes in preparation for your initial interview
- let practice assessor/supervisors and other staff know what learning experiences you would like to do or need to do
- use the opportunities to learn from other healthcare professionals and service users.

Ways of teaching and facilitating learning in practice

There are many ways in which we teach and facilitate learning in practice. In this section, we explore some of these ways and how you might use them to facilitate the learning of others and facilitate your own learning. The NMC (2018) stipulates that as part of our Code of Conduct we must be involved in the learning and development of others and therefore, as students we must start to incorporate this as part of our own development. This section aims to enable you to do this, as well as recognising ways others are supporting your learning and development in practice.

Try this on placement

- Prepare yourself before placement where you can.
- Bring a mini notebook to put in your pocket to write down things you are learning.

- Reflect often and deeply on your experiences using a model.
- Ask questions.
- Make use of the experience around you.
- Seek support from practice assessors, supervisors and academic assessors.
- Most importantly enjoy!

Role modelling

What is it?

A role model is a person worthy of imitating and is viewed as a positive member of a profession. In nursing, research has shown role models are crucial in supporting professional development and assisting students in building confidence and competence in achieving goals in the clinical environment (Jack et al. 2017).

Complete this activity now

Think of a time where you thought a person was a good role model. What did they do? What made them good role models in your view? How did it make you feel?

Complete this activity now

Think of a time when you thought a person was not a good role model. did they do? What made them not good role models in your view? How did it make you feel?

How role modelling can be used as a strategy to teach

Now you have learnt what role modelling is, by providing a good role to others we are showing them the norms and ways to behave and are therefore aiding their learning and developing their professional competence. You have explored what you think makes a good and a poor role model from your own experiences, so you know that there are poor role models; you will see this in placement. However, this can still have a positive impact on your learning and development. By recognising poor behaviours and ways in which you do not what to emulate, this can help you to develop your professional development.

Complete this activity now

How will you be a good role model to others in practice?

Reflective practice

What is reflective practice?

According to the American philosopher Donald Schon, 'Reflective practice is the ability to reflect on one's actions so as to engage in a process of continuous learning' (Schon 1992). Schon refers to reflection in a very simple form, asking us to imagine experiencing the worst week possible and then being offered the opportunity to step into a time machine and return to that bad week to consider and change behaviour relating to what went wrong and your actions around what went right.

The University of Edinburgh Reflection Toolkit (2022) defines reflection as:

> the conscious examination of past experiences, thoughts, and ways of doing things. Its goal is to surface learning about oneself and the situation, and to bring meaning to it in order to inform the present and the future. It challenges the status quo of practice, thoughts, and assumptions and may therefore inform our decisions, actions, attitudes, beliefs, and understanding about ourselves.

University of Edinburgh (2022)

Reflective practice is where we analyse and evaluate an area of our practice or experience to help us to think about the 'what', 'so what' and 'now what' of a given situation. Reflection is a process that most adult human beings experience, but in reflective practice as clinicians we use tools and models to help us to order our thought and flow in doing so.

Why do we reflect?

Reflection helps us to learn through experiencing situations and encounters within the clinical environment, as well as other areas of our lives. It helps us to recognise our thoughts, feelings, strengths and weaknesses in practice and how these might be improved. Reflection assists us to use evidence-based practice in our day-to-day work as clinicians.

How do we reflect?

It should be noted that there are multiple reflective models for clinical practice, the use of which is based on personal preference, as well the situation they can be used in (e.g. clinical work, teaching and presenting).

As you climb through the ranks of your nursing career, you will become more aware of these differing models and how they can be best used. Clinical reflection can be broken down into parts, which as a student you may find more useful. Reflection can take place while in the middle of an experience, although it may feel difficult at first to do this and then post the experience when there may be more down time to reflect on what has taken place during an encounter.

Use of reflective models

As referred to above, clinical reflection models are wide ranging and multiple. However, one of the most useful models used when commencing into learning is the Holm and Stephenson (1994) model of reflection, which has been adapted since its inception. This reflective model is highlighted in Box 5.3.

Box 5.3 | Holm and Stephenson's Reflective Model

Ask yourself:

- What was my role in this situation? (Remembering this is from the perspective of your nursing practice.)
- Did I feel comfortable or uncomfortable? Why?
- What actions did I take?
- How did others and I act?
- Was it appropriate?
- How could I have improved the situation for myself, for others?
- What can I change in the future? Did I feel as if I have learnt anything new about myself?
- Did I expect anything different to happen? What and why?
- Has it changed my ways of thinking in any way?
- What knowledge from theory and research can I apply to this situation?
- What broader issues (e.g. cultural, ethical, legal, political or social) arise from this situation? What do I think about these broader issues?

See one, do one, teach one: the medical training model

What is it?

The 'see one, do one, teach one' training method can be linked back to medical surgical training for medical students, especially those in surgical medicine. The ethos of the model is where the student observes a skill, then is expected to be able to perform a skill and then can teach the skill. It can be related to Kolb's learning theory of learning through experience and doing.

How is it used in practice?

Healthcare professionals, especially those facilitating the learning of others in practice, may use this method by demonstrating a skill in which they are competent to another person. They will then observe other the person undertaking the skill. Once competent, that person can then teach the skill to another.

Try this on placement

- When faced with a new skill, ask your practice assessor/supervisors if you can observe the skill a few times before you do the skill.
- After observing, undertake the skill being observed by your practice assessor/supervisor.
- Once confident in undertaking the skill yourself, have a go at teaching another person how to do the skill.
- Seek feedback throughout.

Summary

The importance of reflection on practice and in practice has been discussed in this section. This section has introduced reflective models and they can be used to enhance learning.

Mentoring/supervision

You learn from other chapters in this book (see, for example, Chapter 8) about how support in practice is achieved through mentoring via a practice assessor and practice supervisor. This section explores how you can get the most out of this support during practice placements.

Understanding from the beginning that your practice assessors and supervisors are there to facilitate and enhance your learning, but without knowing what your own personal learning needs and outcomes are, makes this process extremely difficult to enhance and facilitate. It is important, therefore, for students to have an understanding about their own learning needs and to discuss them with their practice assessor and practice supervisor. This is done during the initial, midpoint and final interviews; however, it can be continuous.

Mentoring and supervision are also linked to role modelling and coaching. Your practice assessor and supervisors will be showing you how to perform as a nurse, supporting you to develop your nursing practice and professionalism, providing you with feedback, and providing you with opportunities to reflect on your performance and to develop. However, to gain the most out of them, we the learner must ask for feedback, use the learning opportunities available, and reflect on our practice where possible to enhance our own learning and development.

Green flag

- Pick appropriate times to discuss learning needs with your supervisor.
- At the start of shifts, let others know what skills you would like to undertake.
- Be specific on what feedback you would like to gain from your supervisors.
- Reflect often on a variety of experiences and take the opportunity to reflect with your supervisor where possible.

Summary

Throughout this chapter, we have explored aspects of learning in practice. We have discussed where and how learning may take place in practice, what types of learning opportunities could be available and how you can maximise learning and development for yourself and how you can enhance the development of others. However, it is essentially you who is the master of how much you maximise your own learning in practice experience.

With the abundance of opportunities available to you to learn in practice it may seem overwhelming. Therefore, being organised and planning and managing your placement time is essential. Throughout, the 'green flag' boxes offer practical tips, providing you with various ways in which to help you to plan and manage your time.

References

Berwick, D. (2013). *A Promise to Learn, a Commitment to Act: Improving the Safety of Patients in England*. Department of Health and Social Care www.gov.uk/government/publications/berwick-review-into-patient-safety (accessed 20 December 2022).

Bubb, S. (2014) Winterbourne View – Time for Change: Transforming the commissioning of services for people with learning disabilities and/or autism. www.england.nhs.uk/wp-content/uploads/2014/11/transforming-commissioning-services.pdf (accessed 20 December 2022).

Faithfull-Byrne, L. et al. (2017). Clinical coaches in nursing and midwifery practice: facilitating point of care workplace learning and development. *Collegian* 24 (4): 403–410. https://doi.org/10.1016/j.colegn.2016.06.001.

Fernandez, E. (1997). Just doing the observations: reflective practice in nursing. *British Journal of Nursing* 6: 16. https://doi.org/10.12968/bjon.1997.6.16.939.

Frances, R. (2013). *Report of the Mid Staffordshire NHS Foundation Trust Public Inquiry. HC 947*. London: Stationery Office https://assets.publishing.service.gov.uk/government/uploads/system/uploads/attachment_data/file/279124/0947.pdf.

Health Education England (2017). www.hee.nhs.uk/our-work/allied-healthprofessions/helping-ensure-essential-supply-ahps/placement-expansion-innovation/resources (accessed 21 February 2023).

Hill, R., Woodward, M., and Arthur, A. (2020). Collaborative learning in practice (CLIP): evaluation of a new approach to clinical learning. *Nurse Education Today* 85: 104295. https://doi.org/10.1016/j.nedt.2019.104295.

Holm, D., and Stephenson, S., (1994). Reflection – A Student's Perspective. In Palmer, A., Burns, S., and Bulman, C. (eds), *Reflective Practice in Nursing: the growth of the professional practitioner*. Blackwell Scientific Publications: Oxford 53–62.

Huggins, D. (2016). Enhancing nursing students' education by coaching mentors. *Nursing Managment* 23 (1): 30–32. https://doi.org/10.7748/nm.23.1.30.s28.

Hughes, S. and Quinn, F. (2013). *Quinn's Principles and Practice of Nurse Education*, 6e. Singapore: Cengage.

Jack, K., Hampshire, C., and Chambers, A. (2017). The influence of role models in undergraduate nursing. *Journal of Clinical Nursing* 26 (23–24): 4707–4715. https://doi.org/10.1111/jocn.13822.

Keogh, B. (2013). Review into the Quality of Care and Treatment Provided by 14 Hospital Trusts in England: Overview report. NHS England. www.basw.co.uk/system/files/resources/basw_85333-2_0.pdf (accessed 16 March 2023).

Nursing and Midwifery Council (2018). Code: Professional Standards of Practice and Behaviour for Nurses, Midwives and Nursing Associates. www.nmc.org.uk/standards/code (accessed December 2020).

Nursing and Midwifery Council (2019). What must be in place. www.nmc.org.uk/supporting-information-on-standards-for-student-supervision-and-assessment/learning-environments-and-experiences/designing-reviewing-safe-effective-learning-experiences/what-must-be-in-place (accessed 20 July 2022).

Schon, D. (1992). *Reflective Practice Toolkit*. University of Cambridge https://libguides.cam.ac.uk/reflectivepracticetoolkit/whatisreflectivepractice (accessed 16 March 2023).

University of Edinburgh (2022) Reflection Toolkit. www.ed.ac.uk/reflection (accessed 6 October 2022).

Whitmore, J. (2017). *Coaching for Performance: The Principles and Practice of Coaching and Leadership*, 5e. London: Nicholas Brealey.

Williamson, G.R., Plowright, H., Kane, A. et al. (2020). Collaborative learning in practice: a systematic review and narrative synthesis of the research evidence in nurse education. *Nurse Education in Practice* 43: 102706. https://doi.org/10.1016/j.nepr.2020.102706.

Willis, P. (2012). *Quality with Compassion: The Future of Nursing Education. Report of the Willis Commission*. Royal College of Nursing https://cdn.ps.emap.com/wp-content/uploads/sites/3/2012/11/Willis-Commission-report-2012.pdf (accessed 3 April 2022).

Willis, P. (2015). *Raising the Bar. Shape of Caring: A Review of the Future Education and Training of Registered Nurses and Care Assistants*. Health Education England https://www.hee.nhs.uk/sites/default/files/documents/2348-Shape-of-caring-review-FINAL.pdf (accessed 21 January 2022).

CHAPTER 6

Getting ready for practice

Mariama Seray-Wurie

AIM

This chapter presents the reader with guidance on how to prepare in advance for the practice learning experience as a student nurse.

LEARNING OUTCOMES

Having read this chapter, the reader will be able to:

1. Discuss what practice learning is and the key processes involved.
2. Demonstrate an awareness of the key requirements for the practice learning experience.
3. Outline strategies to help you prepare for your placement learning.
4. Discuss the importance of looking after your health and wellbeing.

Succeeding on your Nursing Placement: Supervision, Learning and Assessment for Nursing Students, First Edition. Edited by Ian Peate.
© 2024 John Wiley & Sons Ltd. Published 2024 by John Wiley & Sons Ltd.

Introduction

Previous chapters in this book have given you an overview of the role and function of the Nursing and Midwifery Council (NMC), the Standards of Proficiency for Registered Nurses (2018a), Standards of Proficiency for Nursing Associates (NMC 2018b), and an overview of how a programme of study is constructed. Practice learning accounts for 50% of a nursing programme. The clinical placements that students will undertake as part of the nursing programme are an essential part of the process for practice learning that will contribute to the completion of your qualification and becoming an NMC registrant to practice as a nurse or nursing associate. This chapter discusses the importance of practice learning, key requirements and how to prepare ahead for the practice learning experience.

Practice learning

Learning in clinical practice is essential for you to become proficient for your chosen field of practice as set out by the NMC (2018a) at the point of registration as a pre-registration nursing student and for a pre-registration nursing associate student to deliver safe and effective care as detailed by the NMC (2018b). To achieve this proficiency, you will learn by actively engaging in nursing practice (both the art and the science of nursing care). The aim of practice learning is to provide you with the opportunities to achieve the NMC proficiencies, gain knowledge, skills and the attributes for a safe and effective practitioner (NMC 2018c). It should also embody in you an immense sense of curiosity. Practice learning will take place mainly in clinical practice, which will provide the opportunity for you to give direct patient care; however, your nursing programme may deliver some of this learning through simulated practice learning. All the practice learning experiences will equip you with the skills required to become a successful nurse and will include experiences that have an interdisciplinary and interprofessional learning context. One of the key requirements for practice learning is to ensure that, as a student, you are given the opportunity to learn and provide care in a range of clinical settings to ensure that you can meet your programme outcomes and experience care situations for a diverse population. The types of clinical settings you will gain these learning experiences will include:

- hospitals
- community and primary care settings
- other independent health, and social care settings, such as:

- nursing homes
- hospices
- special schools
- prisons.

You may also undertake what is known as a 'hub-and-spoke placement'. Thomas and Westwood (2016) describe this approach as placements being organised to one 'hub' placement per year for placement learning, with the student returning to the hub on three separate occasions throughout the year for blocks of placement. To further enhance learning the student will be allocated a 'spoke' placement, which is linked to the speciality of the hub and reflective of the patient journey across healthcare settings. The 'spoke' placement can last between one and four weeks. A hub-and-spoke placement will provide you with the opportunity to work with healthcare professionals and non-healthcare professionals, depending on the setting, to develop the knowledge and skills and attitude for your field of practice and to achieve the requisite proficiencies.

Over to you

- What do you understand by the term 'lone working'?
- What precautions must you take when lone working?

Read this guide produced by the Royal College of Nursing: www.rcn.org.uk/professional-development/publications/pub-005716

Go online

The practice learning experience is managed by your university in collaboration with practice partners and will be relevant for your field of practice.

- Access the internet and your own university intranet. Identify key staff in your university who are responsible for practice placements. What are their roles and responsibilities.
- Who are the placement partners that your university engages with?

As a student, when you are learning in the clinical practice environment you will be supervised, as it is a requirement that all students are supervised while learning in practice (NMC 2018c); however, the level of supervision required will reflect your learning needs, stage of learning and the placement. The level of supervision that will be given to a first-year student, for example, may be a lot more in comparison with a second- or third-year student. The learning environment may dictate the level of supervision required (e.g. environments such as operating theatres or intensive care units) owing to the nature of the patients and level of care that they require. A practice supervisor will undertake this supervision. This is usually a registered nurse or registered nursing associate who has been prepared to undertake the role as a supervisor of students. There may be times when your practice supervisor is not a registered nurse as they will be a different registered healthcare professional depending on the type of environment in which you are undertaking the practice learning experience. The NMC (2018c) does permit supervision of students by other registered healthcare professionals. They must, however, be registered with a professional regulator; for example, the General Medical Council (GMC) or Health and Care Professions Council (HCPC).

Learning activity 1

Think of examples of other healthcare professionals registered with either the GMC or HCPC. Write a list. In what type of clinical learning environments do you think you may be supervised by another healthcare professional?

(There is a guided answer at the end of the chapter.)

Although the NMC specifies that you need to be supervised by a practice supervisor who is a registered healthcare professional, there may be some practice learning experiences where you are working with non-registered health and social care professions, such as healthcare assistants, maternity support workers or schoolteachers. The role that they will play in your learning will depend on what skill you are required to learn, the experience and skills of the professional and the environment where the learning is to take place. An example situation where you may experience this could be a placement such as a special school, or you may be asked to work with an experienced healthcare assistant to give fundamental nursing care to a patient. These experiences will not be the basis of the whole placement learning experience but they will contribute to the practice learning experience as these non-registered health professions have a wealth of knowledge, skills and experiences that will contribute to your learning on your journey to becoming a registered nurse or nursing associate.

Write here

The professionalism of nurses has always been key to the provision of effective care. However, there has never been a single definition for what it means to act professionally in nursing. Make some notes about what you think professionalism means and then read *Enabling Professionalism in Nursing and Midwifery*: www.nmc.org.uk/globalassets/sitedocuments/other-publications/enabling-professionalism.pdf

Are there any similarities in the notes that you have made and the content in the link provided?

You must be aware, when learning in practice, that you are not accountable, as you have not yet become a registered nurse or nursing associate but you will be responsible for your actions as a student. Part of the theoretical learning about professionalism on your programme would have included learning about the NMC Code (NMC 2018d), which represents the professional standards that all nurses, midwives and nursing associates must uphold if they want to be registered to practise in the UK. The Code is discussed in Chapter 1.

Green flag

As a student, all your practice learning is underpinned by the NMC Code as you are working towards becoming a registered nurse and it is therefore important that you understand how it applies to you now as a student and in your future role as a registered nurse.

Learning activity 2

- What is your understanding of the term 'accountability'?
- How is this different to being 'responsible'?
- Can you think of an example to explain how this applies to you as a student?

(There is a guided answer at the end of the chapter.)

As stated, you are not yet an accountable practitioner, but you are responsible for your actions and therefore as a student you should not participate in any procedures that you do not feel prepared to undertake or confident to do without being adequately supervised. You will find that, as you progress through your programme, the skills and experiences that you will gain from your practice learning experiences will develop and you will become more confident in your abilities to practise safely and with less supervision.

Assessment is the other purpose of undertaking practice learning. Assessment and confirmation of proficiency is a requirement by the NMC. By the end of your programme, for you to become proficient and to demonstrate that proficiency you will need to achieve the relevant proficiencies, skills, and procedures associated with your programme of study. A practice assessor will undertake the assessment of practice. A practice assessor is a registered nurse, midwife or nursing associate who has responsibility for assessing student's practice learning during the period the student is allocated to the clinical placement to confirm of achievement of the proficiencies and programme outcomes. The practice assessor will have had preparation and support to take up their role. They will be knowledgeable about the proficiencies and the outcomes for your programme and stage of learning, which will enable them to undertake an objective, evidence-based assessment of your achievement of the relevant proficiencies, skills and procedures. They will work collaboratively with your practice supervisor to support your learning and decide the outcome of the assessment, which is a continuous process, as a decision will not be made based on a one-off performance of the proficiencies or skills. This means that when you are on placement you will have a named practice assessor and a named practice supervisor as it is a requirement by the NMC that these roles are undertaken by two different people for the period of assessment on the placement.

Over to you

How will find advice and support (if needed) while you are working in placement that is geographically isolated?

Your practice assessor is also responsible for upholding public protection when assessing you and will need to be aware of any concerns regarding your practice and ensure that they take steps to improve your performance and support your learning.

Try this on placement

When in your next clinical placement, make list of the staff with whom you come into regular contact (do not include any nurses). What does your list look like? Did you remember to include all those staff who are absolutely key to supporting services, such as porters, housekeeping staff, pathology staff, ward clerks and so forth. Choose of member of the team and find out as much as you can about their role and their responsibilities.

You will complete a range of practice placement experiences for each part of the programme, which will usually be arranged by your university. Your university will have determined in the curriculum at which point a recommendation for your progression can be made and this is what is known as the progression point. The progression point is when you progress from one part of the programme to the next part. For most nursing programmes, this would usually be at the end of each academic year. At the end of each part, you will need to demonstrate that you are meeting the requirements in practice to progress to the next part or in your final year that you have met the practice requirements to become an NMC registrant. The recommendation for you to progress will be confirmed by your practice assessor and a nominated academic assessor. Academic assessors like practice assessors must be registered nurses, midwives or nursing associates who have been prepared to undertake this role. The academic assessor and practice assessor work in partnership to make these decisions about your progression on the programme with regards to assessment of practice learning. Both practice and academic assessors contribute equally to the progression point decisions, as the practice assessor will have the responsibility to complete the overall assessment of practice and the academic assessor will have insight into your achievements and performance in clinical practice, as well as theoretical learning as the role of the academic assessor is usually a nurse academic from the university. The purpose of this collaborative way of confirming your progression is to ensure that the process is fair and objective taking into consideration theory and practice.

Learning activity 3

Now that you have an overview of the purpose of practice learning, take time out to reflect on the distinct roles of those who will be involved in supporting and assessing your learning in clinical practice. Think about how you can optimise your learning when you are in placement and what support you feel you will need from your practice assessor and practice supervisor.

(There is no guided answer for this reflective point but in Chapter 7 there is further exploration of how you can get the most out of the practice experience and Chapter 8 explores in more detail supervision and assessment; this chapter gives a brief overview in the context of the purpose of practice learning and getting ready.)

Key requirements prior to going into placement

As it has been established that 50% of time on the course will involve learning in practice, this next section focuses on getting you ready for practice and includes pre-reading, contacting and finding out about the placement. Student placement preparation is key for the transition from classroom learning to learning in practice, which was discussed in Chapter 5.

Over to you

Reflect on the content of your theoretical learning experiences to date at the university. How do you think what you have been learning so far will prepare you for the practice learning experience?

Your practice learning experience will commence with preparation for practice. From your reflection, you should have established that the learning experiences at the university will be contributing to this preparation to ensure that you are safe and also prepared as best as possible for the forthcoming experience. There will be some statutory and mandatory training requirements for you to have completed before you can commence placement for the first time and then these must be completed on an annual basis as you progress on the course. Statutory training is compulsory for all employees, as it is training prescribed by a statute of law, and mandatory training is also compulsory training for all employees to support safe delivery of services and ensure the safety and wellbeing of individual staff and patients. Although you are not an employee, as a student you will be involved in direct patient care when learning in practice and therefore your personal health, safety and wellbeing is paramount, as is that of the patients; it is part of the practice learning partnerships between your university and the placement providers that the university ensures that you have completed this learning before you attend placement. These mandatory requirements are outlined in Box 6.1 and are topics that all staff working in health and social care settings complete annually. You will complete these topics via e-learning sessions, as well as completing practical sessions related to some of the topics in the clinical skills centre where you learn your practical skills. Your university will show you how to access the e-learning programme depending on your region in the UK.

As stated earlier in this chapter, the university is responsible for organising your placements. The general principles when allocating your placements will be the programme outcomes, your field of practice and stage of study, as well as other personal circumstances; for example, where you live, if you have access to a car (or other form of personal

Box 6.1 | Statutory and mandatory training

- Conflict resolution
- Data security awareness
- Equality, diversity, and human rights
- Fire safety
- Health, safety and welfare
- Infection prevention and control
- Moving and handling
- Preventing radicalisation: basic prevent awareness
- Resuscitation
- Safeguarding children
- Safeguarding adults
- Reducing risks of violence and aggression

transportation) and whether you have dependants may be taken into consideration. Your university will try as much as possible to factor in your personal circumstances, but you do have to appreciate that it may not always be possible to place you in a clinical area that will meet all your personal requirements as you need to fulfil the requirements of the programme. Part of the practice learning as a student requires you to 'experience the variety of practice expected of registered nurses to meet the holistic needs of people of all ages' (NMC 2018a, 3.2, p. 10) and this will include shift working including some night duty, weekends and bank holidays as care is delivered across 24 hours.

Write here

Think about how you are going to prepare for working shifts if this is something you have never experienced before. What issues could arise and how might you address them?

Having reflected on how you are going to prepare for working shifts, it will be useful for you to revisit your university practice learning handbook. The practice learning handbook has been written to provide you with the key information and guidance to help you through your practice learning journey on the programme. It will outline the key policies and procedures for your university. This document is also shared with the practice learning partners to ensure that they are familiar with your university processes.

Green flag

The practice learning handbook is a document that you will need to return to throughout the programme and definitely at the start of each academic year as policies may have changed or been updated.

The other documents that you will need to familiarise yourself with for the first placement on your programme is the practice assessment document (PAD). This is discussed in more depth in Chapter 9; however, as part of the preparation for practice, your university will run a session on how you are assessed in practice and how to use the PAD. For many universities now, this document is an electronic document and you will need to know your log in details and how to navigate the electronic document. One of the advantages of having an electronic PAD is that you can access the document at any time, minimising the risk of you losing the document or it becoming damaged. It is also timely to have these documents accessible electronically, as many of the practice placement areas in the NHS and some of the independent health and social care providers use electronic patient records and you will be using digital technology to manage patient data.

Hear it from the student

When we where first introduced to the ePAD, I thought there is no way I will ever get the hang of this. It was all so complex. However, one of the other students said to me, 'if you can do your shopping online or order a pizza on line, then there is no reason why you can't use the ePAD' and true enough she was spot on. All it took was just getting used to the platform and having courage! Using the ePAD on a daily basis has really encouraged me and made me much more confident.

Cally, first year mental health student

Your university will inform you of your placement allocation via your clinical placement office or via a web-based software system. Once you know where you will be going to on placement you can start to prepare for that placement specifically. The clinical placement will be your opportunity to put into practice the skills that you have been taught during university teaching weeks and to start working towards becoming proficient. You want to ensure that you are prepared as best as you can, and your university may also deliver further sessions to prepare you for practice before you start. At these sessions, you will be made aware of how to contact your allocated placement, source transport links to the placement and take up a good opportunity to ask questions regarding your learning in practice and the assessment of clinical practice. The session may also include discussions on how to manage external factors related to your wellbeing which are discussed in the final part of this chapter.

In addition to the university preparation, the placement provider (for example, the NHS hospital trust) will invite you to a trust induction day. The induction session is usually led by the clinical placement facilitator for nursing students in the education team for the NHS trust. The induction is an opportunity for the trust to familiarise you with the placement setting and relevant policies to ensure your safety in the first instance such as shift times, breaks, catering facilities and how you will be supported while undertaking placement with the trust. The trusts usually run this day as a virtual event using a web platform since the COVID-19 pandemic but do check as there is a possibility that this could be an in-person event, which will also provide an opportunity to travel to your allocated placement.

Irrespective of a trust induction day, you will need to contact the specific placement area prior to starting the placement, as you may not have the opportunity on the induction day to contact the care area where you have been allocated. The contact details for the area and the specific member of staff such as the ward manager will be in the information you received about the placement allocation. The reason for contacting the ward manager is to introduce yourself to the team, find out what shifts you will be working, who your nominated practice assessor and practice supervisor are, and also to find out a bit more about the ward, clinic or unit. If you have any specific requirements for a shift, this will also be an opportunity to discuss them with the manager. When it comes to the shifts, remember that the clinical placement is your opportunity to gain experience, so you do need to be flexible. The ward manager in many instances would have planned your shifts to ensure that you are working with your supervisor or practice assessor and in some clinical areas they may plan the learning experience to ensure that you rotate through different areas within that clinical setting, have opportunities to work with other healthcare professionals and staff and gain different learning experiences, insight and new perspectives. If you are unable to be flexible with your shift patterns you may lose out on learning opportunities and working with your practice supervisor or practice assessor, and this may impact on the opportunity for your practice assessor to undertake assessment of your practice. Do discuss this with your practice supervisor or practice assessor if this may be an issue.

A supervisor's point of view

One of the best parts of my job is being able to work with student nurses. We love having students in our general practice; they keep us on our toes. We have put together a student orientation pack and this is available to the students about two weeks before they come to us so that they can familiarise themselves with general practice as it is often the first time the student has been allocated to a GP surgery. Students are also encouraged to go online and look at our practice website. Again, this gives them a little more insight in to what we are all about at Scammel Street Surgery.

I would always recommend to any student to make contact with the placement before they are due to start. This will give them a heads up, easing them into the care area in more gentle way.

Miranda, practice nurse

Most placement areas will have a orientation pack. An orientation pack helps learners to understand the area, the types of patients/service users they will be involved with in direct care, the care areas' underpinning philosophy of care, a glossary of abbreviations, and may include some pre-learning for you to undertake prior to your commencing the placement. It is particularly useful to have this information ahead of you starting your shifts as it will contribute to your preparation. Even if there is no pre-learning or you have not been given an orientation pack, still find out about the speciality and types of patients/service users for that area and make sure that you do some background research and reading from relevant peer reviewed journals for the speciality. You can also refer to what you have been learning in theory and how this knowledge will be applied when on placement as it is key that you do not see that what you have learned in theory as separate from what you will be learning in practice.

Once you have some knowledge of the type of learning experience and patient/service users you will be giving direct or indirect care to, you can start to think about setting some learning objectives for the placement to discuss with your practice assessor when you start. Learning objectives are what will define your learning in terms of development and achievement during the practice learning experience and having an idea of what you want to achieve shows that you have thought about your learning, what you can achieve and prepare for your initial interview as part of the assessment of practice. You may find this difficult to do at first or think you may have done it wrong. However, remember that when you start the placement you will be able to discuss your thoughts on what you would like to achieve with your practice assessor who will then give you guidance to ensure that what you want to do is realistic and achievable.

By investing time in how you prepare for your practice learning experience through attendance at preparation for practice, trust inductions and arranging a pre-placement visit or telephone call with the ward manager demonstrates that you are being proactive in your learning and students who do well in placement tend be pro-active and open to anything they might learn (NHS n.d.)

Complete this activity now

Getting ready for practice scenarios

Outlined are three distinct types of placement scenarios that are not the usual hospital-based placement. Consider how you would personally prepare yourself for each placement.

Scenario 1

You have received your first placement allocation and you will be spending six weeks in a nursing care home that specialises in dementia care and end of life dementia care.

Scenario 2

Your placement allocation is in the primary care setting. You have been allocated to a placement in general practice and will be working Monday through to Friday in a GP surgery for eight weeks.

Scenario 3

You have been allocated to a special needs school for students aged 16–24 years of age for one week as part of a hub-and-spoke placement In the community with the community learning disability team and school nurses.

(There is a guided answer at the end of the chapter with useful resources.)

Your health and wellbeing

This section of the chapter addresses how to manage your health, wellbeing and expectations as this is an important aspect of your life as a student nurse, and particularly when you embark on your first placement learning experience, if you have never had any exposure to working in healthcare. Brady et al. (2019) considered the first practice placement experience of children's nursing students. They identified that the first practice placement is of utmost importance in confirming the choice of a student to study nursing. In their review of the literature, they identified that the first placement can cause anxiety, stress and uncertainty for students. This is a view that is supported by Grobecker (2016) and Levett-Jones et al. (2015) identifying in their studies that the anxiety about placement learning and the reality of nursing is a concern locally, nationally and internationally. Preparation for the practice learning experience can help in alleviating some of these anxieties before you go to placement and offer further guidance while you are on placement.

While you are on placement, you will need to participate in direct care of patients and undertake shift work and this may be the first time you are doing shift work or even if you have worked in healthcare the shifts may be different to how you have been used to working. There is also the addition of keeping up to date with your academic work while on placement as theory and practice are linked and it is important for you not to see the two types of learning as separate.

In summary, the role of being a student nurse can be stressful, as the clinical placements at times can be demanding; as an individual you are juggling different competing demands and therefore it is important to learn how to take care of yourself.

> ## Reflective activity
>
> Take time out to think about how you are feeling about your upcoming clinical placement and any anxieties or fears that you may have about going to placement. You may want to discuss these feelings with your personal tutor or at your preparation for practice sessions when in university.

The feelings that you may have, such as excitement, fear and anxiety, are all normal, as these are emotions that most people – even outside nursing – would experience when embarking on something that they have never done before or that is different to what they have been used to. What you do not want is the fear and anxiety to hinder your practice learning when you start the placement. The reflective activity earlier asked you to identify any anxiety or fears, now what you can do with your list is to divide the fears and anxieties into external factors to help you take a proactive approach to managing expectations. Being proactive means that you will be in control of your situation. External factors causing anxiety may be things such as travelling to the placement and the cost of travelling, worrying that you may not eat properly, or having to submit assessments while on placement. These external factors are things that you can take control of and manage. Examples of how you can manage the identified external factors are by using your university student services to ensure that you are claiming all the support you are entitled to as student nurse, such as the additional amount of money per year that can help with living costs as a home student, using your course academic planner and assessment map, and discussing with the ward manager how you can manage your shifts to ensure that you can have some time to complete and submit your assessments.

Over to you

If you are required to work night duty, put together a list that will help you to prepare for your first night shift.

- What does sleep deprivation mean to you and how might it impact on the care that you deliver?

For those fears and anxieties that are not caused by external factors, the emotions that you are not able to control, such as performance anxiety, fear of caring for dying patients, fear of not being able to socialise into the clinical environment, fear of COVID-19, these are issues that you would need to use the support systems before and during your placement. You can talk about these fears with your personal tutor before you start placement, although the study undertake by Levett-Jones et al. (2015) found that by attempting to alleviate the anxiety expressed by some students before the first placement through preparation for practice may be counterproductive and increase the anxiety and therefore may hinder the student's ability to function effectively. As an alternative approach, Levett-Jones et al. (2015) suggest that the supervisors of practice need to address the student's emotional needs helping them to build on their pre-existing skills of what they know and can do thus, empowering the student to succeed. This suggests that within the practice learning environment there needs to be a culture of nurturing for the student's first learning experience. Your practice supervisor and your practice assessor will have a key role in supporting you on placement, as will having peer support during the placement. In addition to your peers, the supervisors and assessors, your university will also have staff who support learning in practice such as link lecturers or clinical teachers who are also a source of support if you are experiencing difficulties and will be able to sign post you to the appropriate support services within the university.

It may be that you do not have any anxieties, but you still have to be able to take care of your health and wellbeing and plan how you will manage things such as getting enough rest and sleep, eating properly and staying healthy. This is when the wellbeing services within your university are able to suggest resources with strategies to help you develop the student/placement/work life balance.

To help you focus on getting ready for practice, Box 6.2 has a checklist that identifies the key points for getting ready. Chapter 7 builds on this chapter with a focus on getting the most out of practice from the student perspective.

Box 6.2 | Things to do to ensure that you are ready for placement

- Complete all your mandatory training? (See Box 6.1 and refer to your university practice learning handbook.)
- If you have received your placement allocation, find out about the specific practice placement profile through the range of resources available to you, which may include practice profiles and the trust's website.
- Attend the preparation for practice sessions and trust Inductions.
- Familiarise yourself with the PAD and learn how to navigate the document if it is digital.
- Contact the practice placement area at least two weeks in advance of starting to introduce yourself, discuss shift patterns, know who your nominated practice assessor and practice supervisor are.
- Undertake a trial run to the placement area so that you can plan your travel time.
- Undertake some background reading about the clinical speciality and types of patient/service users that you will be involved in the management of their care.
- Other documents to read: the Code, Guidance on raising concerns, Guidance on using social media, Guidance on

the professional duty of candour and Enabling professionalism (accessible from the NMC website).

- Be proactive and set some learning objectives before you start, as you should have knowledge of the type of learning experience you will be having.
- Have you got your uniform and appropriate footwear? If you are not required to wear a uniform, do you know what the dress code policy is for the placement area?
- Look after your physical health as well and remember to get adequate sleep to and to eat properly.
- Develop a positive mental attitude and be open to the learning experiences.

Summary

An essential part of any nursing programme are the practice placements. They prepare you with the skills that you will need for a successful nursing career. All nursing students take on supernumerary status when on placement. While on clinical placement (50% of course time), many opportunities will arise that will enable you to apply theoretical learning into clinical practice.

Prior to attending clinical placement, learn as much as you can about the area. Always make contact with the care area you are being allocated to and introduce yourself. There are a number of people on placement and at the university who can offer you support so you are able to get the most out of the learning experience. Do not struggle in silence, raise any concerns you may have. It is important to remember, that you are in your clinical placement to learn and develop a deeper understanding of this complex and fascinating thing that is called nursing.

References

Brady, M., Price, J., Bolland, R., and Finnerty, G. (2019). Needing to belong: first practice placement experiences of children's nursing students. *Comprehensive Child and Adolescent Nursing* 42 (1): 24–39.

Grobecker, P.A. (2016). A sense of belonging and perceived stress among baccalaureate nursing students in clinical placements. *Nurse Education Today* 16: 178–183.

Levett-Jones, T., Pitt, V., Courtenay-Pratt, H. et al. (2015). What are the primary concerns of nursing students as they prepare for and contemplate their first clinical placement experience? *Nurse Education in Practice* 15: 304–309.

NHS (n.d.). Your first placement. www.healthcareers.nhs.uk/career-planning/study-and-training/considering-or-university/support-university/your-first-placement (accessed 5 November 2022).

Nursing and Midwifery Council (2018a). *Realising Professionalism: Standards for Education and Training. Part 3: Standards for Pre-registration Nursing Programmes.* London: NMC www.nmc.org.uk/Programme-standards-nursing (accessed 16 March 2023).

Nursing and Midwifery Council (2018b). *Realising Professionalism: Standards for Education and Training: Standards for Pre-registration Nursing Associate Programmes.* London: NMC www.nmc.org.uk/standards/standards-for-nursing-associates (accessed 16 March 2023).

Nursing and Midwifery Council (2018c). The Code: Code: Professional Standards of Practice and Behaviour for Nurses, Midwives and Nursing Associates. www.nmc.org.uk/standards/code (accessed 16 March 2023).

Nursing and Midwifery Council (2018d). *Realising Professionalism: Standards for Education and Training. Part 2: Standards for Student Supervision and Assessment.* London: NMC www.nmc.org.uk/Student-supervision-assessment (accessed 16 March 2023).

Thomas, M. and Westwood, N. (2016). Student experience of hub and spoke model of placement allocation – an evaluative study. *Nurse Education Today* 46: 24–28.

Useful resources

Nursing and Midwifery Council (2023). Guidance and Supporting Information. www.nmc.org.uk/standards/guidance (accessed 16 March 2023).

Royal College of Nursing (2016). Personal Safety When Working Alone: Guidance for Members Working in Health and Social Care. www.rcn.org.uk/professional-development/publications/pub-005716 (accessed 16 March 2023).

Learning activities outline answers

Learning activity 1 Examples of other healthcare professionals that you may work with who can supervise you are general practitioners, social workers, paramedics, physiotherapists, occupational therapists, and operating department practitioners.

The types of placements where you may be supervised by another healthcare professional would be a general practice, walk-in centre or minor injuries unit, rehabilitation centre, operating theatre, community mental health and learning disabilities setting, ambulatory paediatrics, special schools.

Learning activity 2 Accountability and responsibility, concepts that are often intertwined in nursing. Point 11 of the Code: practise safely states, 'Be accountable for your decisions to delegate tasks and duties to other people'. To be accountable is to take responsibility for clinical decisions, actions, and omissions – and to be able to justify your decisions. A registered nurse/nursing associate is professionally accountable to the NMC as a registrant. As a student and not a registrant you are not accountable to the NMC; however, the law does impose a duty of care on you as a student and that duty of care applies when you are involved in any care activities that have been delegated to you by the registered nurse/nursing associate, which is why you are responsible for your actions.

An example of this would be your practice supervisor asking you to undertake a wound dressing in the leg ulcer clinic that involves applying compression bandaging. You know the patient, as you have seen the wound being dressed before. You go ahead and do the dressing and apply a normal bandage not a compression bandage, as you were not aware that there was a difference. This was observed by the healthcare associate in the clinic, who informed your supervisor that you have applied the wrong bandaging. In this scenario, your practice supervisor is accountable as they delegated this task to you; however, you have a duty of care to work proficiently and not to work beyond your level of proficiency, which you did as you were not knowledgeable about the purpose of compression bandaging.

Learning activity 3: getting ready for practice scenarios
Scenario 1 A nursing care home offers a wealth of learning opportunities – in this case, dementia care and end of life dementia care. You can undertake some research about dementia care and end of life dementia care. Identify the care home team are then focus on the role of nurses and nursing associates. You can also find out about interprofessional working and what opportunities there will be for you. If you think that your learning will be limited as you are having a placement in a nursing care home, you should think again, as you will be able to achieve many of the physical assessment proficiencies as well as the communication skills and therapeutic relationships whatever your field of practice. Below is a useful link for a resource about transition to care home nursing by the Queens Nursing Institute: www.qni.org.uk/wp-content/uploads/2018/01/Transition-to-Care-Home-Nursing-Chapter-4.pdf

Scenario 2 A placement in a GP surgery for a period of eight weeks working Monday–Friday may seem like a daunting prospect; however, the delivery of healthcare has shifted from secondary to primary care settings, which means that if the future primary care workforce is to be developed, it is essential that more student nurses have exposure to a range of nursing roles in primary care settings. Again, in this scenario it is important to do some research on the role of general practice and the type of learning experiences you will be exposed to as well as the primary care team that makes up the practice. An example of the team would include GPs, advanced nurse practitioners, general practice nurses, nursing associates and healthcare assistants, as well as the administrative staff. A general practice will also work in partnership with other health professionals such as midwives, district nurses, pharmacists, to name a few. There is usually scope for 'spoke' placements to enhance your learning. You may also think about how the shifts will work across the week.

Scenario 3 A placement in a special needs school for one week. This is an example of how a 'hub-and-spoke' placement works, as the experience is for one week. As it is a special school, it is more than likely you will be working in partnership with the teachers at some point during the week if the school nurse is not present. As mentioned earlier in this chapter, there may be occasions when you will be working with a non-healthcare professional and this is acceptable within the context of the learning opportunity that the experience will offer, so this should not put you off. You will need to have clear focus on what you will want to achieve for that week and how it will contribute to your overall learning with the community learning disability team.

CHAPTER 7

Getting the most out of the practice experience

Sebastian Birch, Laura Wasey, and Serena Khoury

AIM

The aim of this chapter is to provide the reader with insight and information to help them get the most out of their placements.

LEARNING OUTCOMES

Having read this chapter, the reader will be able to:

1. Outline the role and contribution they make as they undertake the placement experience.
2. Understand the importance of gaining insight with regards to the allocated placement prior to arriving.
3. Discuss the benefits of discussing with placement staff what your needs are (e.g. childcare/personal requirements) and any adjustments that may be needed.
4. Demonstrate an awareness and understanding of the need to always act in professional manner while working in the placement area.

Succeeding on your Nursing Placement: Supervision, Learning and Assessment for Nursing Students, First Edition. Edited by Ian Peate.
© 2024 John Wiley & Sons Ltd. Published 2024 by John Wiley & Sons Ltd.

Introduction

In this chapter we look at some hints and tips to help you get the most out of your placements. Two of the contributors to this chapter (LW and SK) are student nurses. This chapter is more informal and will consist mainly of things that I wish I had known when I did my nursing placements, quite a while ago now. There is one formal document that any student nurse (or experienced nurse for that matter) should get familiar with and that is the Nursing and Midwifery Council (NMC) Standards for Student Supervision and Assessment (NMC 2018; see Chapter 8). In this document the NMC sets out its processes for student assessment in placement. In an ideal world, each placement will know this and will be ready for students. However, it might be the case that a placement has been reopened to students, is brand new or has had a changeover of staff who are unfamiliar with the new standards. This could mean that you are not allocated a practice assessor and a practice supervisor as required by the standards (NMC 2018). For you to ask for this support, you need to know what you are asking. I would highly recommend knowing this document and knowing it very well. Refer also to Chapter 6 where further detail is provided about preparation for placement.

My own journey as a student nurse

I would like to give a brief outline of my journey through my student nurse practice experience. I would like to do this for a couple of reasons. Firstly, so that if you are reading this and think 'ppppfffttt, this old timer doesn't know what they are on about!' You will be able to see that we would have been through many of the same emotions leading up to and during placement. Secondly, and probably most importantly, those of you embarking on your first placement to those who are on your last management placement can know that you are not alone. We have all been scared, wanted to ask questions, and felt out of our depth. I am a mental health nurse, I did the postgraduate diploma (which is a condensed two-year course after you have done a previous degree). This meant that our placements and teaching were squashed into two years instead of three. My first placement was on a 20-bedded mixed acute adult ward. I turned up in smart trousers and a shirt (I had no idea). I walked up to the nurse's station; I introduced myself 'Hello, I'm Seb and this is my first placement', proud as punch. The nurse in charge looked at me, eyed me up and down and said 'Your first placement you say? Well, I never would have guessed'. Just then someone comes up to the nurse's station, says they feel a little bit sick and was then very poorly on the floor. I realised instantly that the shirt and trousers were a mistake.

Second placement

My next placement was with an older adult community team. We would visit residents in care homes and talk to the residents who had complex diagnoses and were exhibiting aggressive behaviour. We would talk to the residents and find out what was causing this aggression; not just medicate them. It was an amazing team, delivering psychosocial interventions to prevent the overuse of medication in frail people. I had long hair at the time, which I did not tie up. After a week of my hair being pulled, I tied it up. I then had what felt like 100 community placements in a row. This made me a little disillusioned with placements as I felt that I was repeating myself. I know now, from being on the other the side of placements and working at a university, that there are strict pathways set out by the NMC for each field of nursing that the placement officers must stick to. They are not being mean; they are not being fussy; they are sharing out a small number of placements to a lot of students and making sure that we are all meeting our NMC required pathways. It was my final placement though that I felt like I made the transition from *student* to *nurse*.

Final placement

My final placement was on a 12-bed medium secure forensic unit. It was my management placement, and I was there for three months. I really felt like I knew the staff and the service users. There was one shift I remember. I was coming in on an early shift and I sat in the handover room. There were no substantial members of staff on the day shift. Which meant that the night nurse could not go home until there was someone substantive they could hand the shift over to. I, being young and a bit silly, offered to take the shift over to let the night shift go home. I felt I was ready, I had been there for months, I knew what I was doing. I am so glad that the night shift nurse in charge sat me down and explained to me why that would be a bad idea. Firstly, I was a student. Secondly, I was a student. I believe the third reason was that I was, well, a student. I could not have taken over the shift because it would have been dangerous. So, we waited and called the on-call managers, who came down and relieved the shift. This taught me a few things. Firstly, how important it is to work within your safe capacity. As a student nurse I would not have been able to give medication, use physical restraint or have the experience to run a ward. Secondly, the experience taught me that you need to poke your head out above the parapet to learn. If you are not pushing yourself a little bit, you will not maximise your placement potential. If I had not put myself forward in that situation, I would not have learnt the procedures fully, or known why a student cannot act in that way. Thirdly, how much nursing staff want to teach. I was not shouted at; I was not made to feel ridiculous for asking, I was taught. That has carried on with me throughout my varied career as a nurse.

Green flag

Practice learning is where you will put into place all the distant, difficult and abstract things you learn in university. Practice placement is where you fully become a nurse.

Hints and tips

Before placement

What is the first thing you should do to make the most out of your placement? I would say, it is understanding the area you are going into. You might have been placed in district nursing for the first time and if you turn up on day one without having a rough idea of what that practice area does, you will not be able to maximise your practice learning, because you will always be playing catch up I recommend doing some research into the practice area. Look up the ward/wing/area online to see what their clinical specialty is. Then hit the books. Your university library will have copies (most probably electronic copies) of textbooks on that specific area of nursing. Give these a read; see what skills are used in these areas and compare these with the skills you have already seen. What do you need to learn to excel in this area? Write down a list of everything you would like to see/achieve/learn about in that placement area. Doing your basic research has many advantages for starting placement:

- You will hit the ground running and feel more confident when you start placement.
- You will not have to be asking questions all the time to get up to speed.
- You will show that you are an eager, dedicated, student, and this will mean that busy practice assessors and supervisors will be able to include you in higher level tasks, thus accelerating your learning.

A supervisor's notes

It is always a joy to have students nurses allocated to our clinic. We learn as much from the students as, we hope, they learn from us and our clients and their carers. I know when the student has done some preliminary reading and research prior to coming to us as they understand a little regarding our philosophy of care.

Dora, clinical nurse specialist learning disabilities

It is a good idea to call ahead and introduce yourself. This will achieve a couple of things. First, you will be able to confirm a start time, you will be able to get a name of the person who will be your practice assessor and, most importantly, you will show yourself as an eager learner. I would recommend calling one week before (do not be offended if they do not know you are coming, bring this back to your academic advisor/link lecturer at university). This leaves enough time for any issues to be corrected, but not too much time for your name to be written down and potentially misplaced. When you are making this call, as well as introducing yourself, ask if there is any pre-reading you should do about the placement. You might well be going to a clinical area you have never worked in before, never even heard of in some cases. As such there will be a vast range of knowledge needed for the placement that you might not have had the chance to acquire yet. Asking for suggestions for pre-reading will show how eager you are to learn and equip you with the correct knowledge before you arrive at placement so you can hit the ground running. I recommend asking for:

- Theoretical knowledge you will need (anatomy and physiology).
- Pharmacology you will need to know (what medicines are used in this clinical area, what at the side effects of those medications, what monitoring is needed).

- Legal aspects of the placement (this is important for students of all nursing fields); think for example about the legal implications of nursing people in a care home with diminished capacity.
- Clinical skills you will need to know.

Discuss any childcare/personal requirements and adjustments before arriving (occupational health requirements, other caring requirements). It is important you talk to you practice assessor about these things because there might be reasonable adjustments that can be put in place before you arrive at the placement area. If these are in place, then you are going to be in a much better place to get the most of your placement experience. Remember that this is a clinical area that is meeting the need of patients/service users; do not demand and prepare to be flexible. For example, you might have an idea that you can only start at 0900 hours instead of the shift pattern start of 0720 hours. You might be able to have a discussion around changing your start time a little bit, but this is a clinical area whose primary concern is the care they give to patients, you need to fit within that care. Turning up at 0900 hours every day would mean that you miss the morning handover, allocation and, most likely, the first medication round. This is a lot of clinical experience you will be missing. If the area says no to you changing your hours, then take this on board and react to it respectfully.

Make sure you know the shift pattern for your first week. Ask about the shift patterns the placement area operates on (do not assume from a previous placement). I can remember moving between different NHS trusts (and across private and NHS providers) and there being a dramatic change in shift times. So, make sure you ask for the times in your initial phone call! Also, in my experience, most placement areas will suggest that you work 9 to 5 for the first week, to make sure all the first-week administration is done. However, this will not always be the case, so never assume.

This bit of advice might seem like I am stating the obvious, but make sure you know where you are going. I can remember looking at a map of the first hospital I had my mental health placement on and being utterly confused. The map did not seem to be connected to the actual road layout of the hospital because there was construction work going on. The coloured areas of the map did not actually correlate to the colour codes on all the ward doors. As a final hurdle to jump, some of the doors were not even named or numbered. I remember being very late to my first hand over. One great way to make sure you know where you are going, how long it is going to take, and what the travel conditions are like is to do a practice run at the same time you will be attending placement. That way, if there is traffic on the roads in the morning, or the train station is a little way away from the placement, you know about it and can adjust your travelling plans accordingly.

Think about your lunch/meals. It might be busy so do not bring anything that is too complicated. This might seem obvious, but we need fuel; if you are not eating correctly on placement, you will not be able to concentrate; if you cannot concentrate you will not be able to take in information; if you are not able to take in information you will not be able to make the most out of your practice learning. The same goes for sleep. There is a fine line that needs to be walked between your personal life (i.e. jobs, family, social life) and placement.

During placement

My first piece of advice for starting placement – in fact for all jobs/courses/placements – is to be early. This has many positive points in that you will reduce your own stress levels, and you will not rub the placement area up the wrong way by being late on your first day. I recall a piece of advice given to me by a seasoned charge nurse; I will be paraphrasing, but it went something like this: 'The night shift can only go home if the early shift has turned up and you do not want to see what happens if you annoy a tired night shift'. While on placement, you will be supernumerary (meaning that you will not be counted into the safe staffing numbers); you should still consider yourself to be a member of the team, as such it is a good habit to get into.

Try this on placement

To familiarise yourself with a care area that you have never been allocated to before, do a dummy run. How long will it take you to get there? Where is the area physically located? How do you gain access? and so forth. This may relieve some of the stress and anxiety you may have when arriving for your real first day.

Listen in handover. This is another piece of advice that might seem so obvious its almost insulting to mention. However, handover is one of the most important clinical events of the day, it does not matter which field of nursing you are studying, handover is where you will get all the important information for the day. You will get information on risk, tasks and service user status. I would highly recommend writing notes (especially for new patients/service users) but be very mindful of what you do with these notes as they would be considered confidential information, so remember to put them in the confidential waste bin before you go home.

Ask lots of questions and have a notepad that you can write the answers down in. There is no such thing as a silly question and the more you ask the more you will lean. Ask if there is a 'student pack' – this should have any induction materials in (fire exits, codes for the sluice, and all manner of other info). Saying earlier that there is no such thing as a silly question, there is such a thing as a question covered elsewhere. So do not be upset if your question is redirected to the student pack.

Take initiative and say yes to tasks. Do not wait for your assessor or staff to assign you things to do, go out and seek them. Put yourself out there and ask if you can be involved. This is a trait of successful learning, seeking out new experiences. However, it is always important to remember to practice within your scope of competency. For example, if you are seeing lots of cannulation but are only a first year, first placement student do not be surprised if you are told that performing such a skill is beyond your scope of practice for now. Also do not be upset if you ask to attend a psychology session and it is deemed unsuitable to do so. This could be for many reasons, such as confidentiality or risk. It is always good to ask, but also good to accept a 'no'.

Go to MDT (multidisciplinary team) meetings, sit in on therapeutic groups, engage with patients, talk to other healthcare professionals. One thing I can say with absolute certainty, no matter what field of nursing you are studying, no matter where in the world you are studying it: you will learn more from being on the floor than you will in the nursing office. What do I mean by this? You need to be out and about, interacting with service users, performing clinical skills, and learning from other health care professionals. You will not be maximising your own learning if you are glued to the nurse's station, on your phone, or avoiding clinical duties. You also might find yourself falling into a rut and just carrying out mundane work you have done before (such as restocking or folding laundry). When we fall into these behaviours, we might think of them as ritualistic. There are many reasons why we might be avoidant of clinical tasks; the most common will be anxiety. When nurses (not just nurses but all people) become anxious we fall back onto rituals to reduce our anxiety (Walsh and Ford 1989). We need to be mindful of when these happen (working reflectively will help with this) and push ourselves to break out of ritualistic behaviour. This is especially important for placement learning, because there is no safer or better time to be learning new skills than when you are a student; you have a whole team around you dedicated to your learning, you are not counted in the clinical numbers, and you are allowed all the practice you need.

Discuss your learning objectives with your assessor, discuss things you want to learn and experience and perhaps other clinical areas you would like insight in. It is important for your learning that you speak to your practice assessor in your initial interview and let them know what you would like to get from this practice placement, what you have learnt from previous placements, and if there are any skills outstanding that you will need to complete before the end of the part. This last point is one that is especially important. As I am sure the nursing students reading this are aware, at the end of each part you will need to be signed off by an academic assessor and a practice assessor. For this to happen, you will need to have met all the criteria for the part, one of these criteria is the completion of part specific skills. In my time lecturing, I reminded too many students throughout the year to keep an eye on their part specific skills. I suggest that in every placement you speak to your practice assessor and let them know which skills you have left to complete. There will be some that will be more difficult to complete than others throughout the year. This is especially true for mental health students and some of the more technical skills (nasogastric tube feeding, for example). However, in thinking with your practice assessor you might well be able to come up with outreach placement areas in which you can learn and practice these skills. To do this though, your assessor needs to know what skills you have left to do.

Green flag

Familiarise yourself with the ward, get to know other student nurses to find out what their experience has been.

Speak to your link lecturer/academic advisor or practice education facilitators if there any issues that you feel you cannot speak to your assessor about. There might be things that are placement area specific that you have not encountered before in your journey to be a registered nurse. For example, when I was lecturing, I would stress to adult nursing students that their mental health insight placement would be very different to their usual placement areas, They will see things that they might find uncomfortable (such as restraint), but these things

Box 7.1 | Some phrases that could help you to raise concerns

- I have just seen X, I wonder if you could explain why that happened to me?
- I'm new to this area of practice; please could you explain something I have seen to me?
- Is it best practice to . . .?
- Is there anything I could read about something I saw on shift yesterday . . .?

are necessary to preserve life and are carried out by educated, competent professionals. However, this is context specific. There could be some instances where you see something that could be considered malpractice, or even abuse. If there are any issues to do with malpractice, talk to your practice assessor, practice supervisor, practice education facilitator as soon as possible. I would suggest doing this in an inquisitive manner. Being open and curious about the practice you have seen. See Box 7.1, for some phrases that could help you to raise concerns.

It is important to flag up things you see with your practice assessor as soon as possible after you see them. However, it might be the case that your practice assessor is not on shift or you are not working with them that week. In this case it is important to talk to your practice supervisor for the shift, the ward manager, or your link lecturer from university. This is for one simple reason: if what you saw was dangerous it could be being repeated, and your practice assessor needs to do something to ensure safety. However, there are times that student's report that they feel uncomfortable talking to their practice assessor about issues. In this case it is important to speak to your link lecturer as soon as possible, do not leave it to your next meeting but email them and explain what it is happening. It might be that people's safety is depending on it.

The two Rs

There are two Rs to getting the most out of your placement, these are *resilience* and *reflection*.

Reflection

> It is not sufficient to have an experience in order to learn. Without reflecting on this experience, it may quickly be forgotten, or its learning potential lost.
>
> (Gibbs 1988)

Gibbs makes a powerful argument and it is one we need to heed. Reflecting in nurse education is one of the most important skills we can develop. It makes us better clinicians not only in understanding our own practice and developing it, but also in understanding the lives of our service users. This is all the more important while on practice placements. You will be encountering new skills and new situations, and working within new clinical settings. Some of the events you see you may never have seen before. Without reflecting on these events, sometimes as a group or with your practice assessor and practice supervisor, you will not be able to take the full learning out of the situation. I can remember seeing my first rapid tranquilisation happen when I was a student mental health nurse. Rapid tranquilisation is a clinical procedure used in psychiatry when someone is posing an immediate danger to themselves and/or others when all other modes of de-escalation have been tried or deemed too risky. The procedure involved using medication, sometimes via intramuscular injection, to rapidly reduce agitation. It can sometimes be upsetting to be part of. If I did not have space for reflection with my mentor (this is what practice assessors used to be called) after this incident, I would not have fully understood why it was needed, what steps had gone into de-escalating the situation before we reached the need for rapid tranquilisation and could well have developed a warped view of its need and use. Reflection allows for us to change our attitude and response to events and incidents, helping us grow as clinicians. Coming from the university setting to the practice setting is also something that can be helped by reflection (Schön 1983). This bridging of the theory–practice gap is something that we all need to do as clinicians. This is something that reflection can help with. Let us show the need for reflection in bridging with an example. When training as a mental health nurse, you come across lots of different psychosocial interventions; you also come across lots of different people with lots of different mental health issues. Not all the interventions are going to be suitable for every person. I recall learning how to make a genogram (a type of family tree used in systemic thinking/interventions to look at the relationships between a service user and their wider support/family and friend network). This was exciting because it felt like in the classroom, I was doing the genogram well. I was going on placement in the coming weeks and I had decided that I wanted to work with a service user to create a genogram. I was on placement on a ward and working with a service user as their named nurse, I decided in one of our daily sessions that I would start to conduct a genogram with this client. However, the client was not fully ready to discuss their family and their connections to their family. I tried to persuade the service user to give it a go, but in doing so I really damaged our therapeutic relationship. This was certainly something I needed to reflect on. Through my reflection, I realised that not all interventions were suitable for all people. Some people are at different stages of their recovery and as such are at different stages of being able to speak about their past (especially if their past was traumatic). So, from my reflection, I learnt to not push my therapeutic agenda on to someone and to work with them to deliver the best intervention at the best time. This has stuck with my clinical practice since. I would highly recommend reading a book called *Reflective Practice for Healthcare Professionals* by Taylor (2010). This chapter is too short to have a full exploration into the use of reflection in learning but hopefully by highlighting it you can start to develop your own reflective practice to help. I would not have learnt the things I have learnt on placement when I was a student to the level I learnt them without the reflective element. I would not also be the clinician I am today without reflective practice. It is a skill for all nurses, one that will make you a better nurse.

> ## Over to you
>
> Take some time out from reading this chapter to think of an intervention you were part of on placement that you would like to have done better. It does not need to be a life or death intervention, it can be as big or as small as you like (I think we spend a lot of time reflecting on the big things in practice and leave out the smaller things, so it might well be interesting to pick something small). Then look up the Gibbs reflection model and read over it. Now write out a reflective piece using the steps of the Gibbs model.

When on placement it is important to keep thinking and writing reflectively, not only because these will be needed for your practice assessment document (PAD) or ePAD but also your essays at university will need to have some (Box 7.2; see Chapter 9 of this text for a discussion on the PAD).

Box 7.2 | Reflective practice ideas

- Reflect on what could or did go wrong rather than provide evidence of everything 'going perfectly'. For example, this could be a reflection on a patient interaction or an observation.
- Reflect on an adverse incident in the department. What procedures have been put in place to avoid this from happening again and is there anything else that could be done?
- Reflect on visits to different departments or areas of practice. For example, produce a reflective account of a visit to accident and emergency and of the practices observed there. You could include mind maps and charts in this kind of account.
- Use simulation to generate reflection. Simulations can be useful for events and situations that rarely happen (you will have been doing simulations at university, but it can also be a powerful tool to learn on placement, especially if you are about to deliver a skill in a new environment, you can ask your practice assessor or supervisor if you can perform the skill in a simulated setting before a 'live-fire' setting).
- Write a reflective piece of an event you have attended (if you have been to any training or continuing professional development slot that is run at your placement area).
- With a colleague/fellow student's consent, film a simulated encounter with them and afterwards you can critically reflect on your performance. You could focus on your communication skills and how they might be improved.
- Produce a reflective summary of a discussion with your practice assessor. Consider what was learned from this, that will be put into practice in future events?

Source: Adapted from Health Education England (2021).

Resilience

We know that being a nurse is a difficult yet rewarding profession. We as nurses are some of the professionals who are with people in their darkest hours and their brightest hours. This can be taxing on our own wellbeing. Student nursing and being on placement is no different. You will experience stress, loss and negativity when you are out on your placements. If you are not careful, this can interfere with your own wellbeing and as such with your ability to learn. Therefore, *resilience* is so important for making the most out of your placement learning.

One way to build resilience to is make sure we are looking after our physical, emotional, and spiritual selves. A method of doing this is called *self-care*. Before explaining how to use self-care, we need a moment to explain why it is useful for getting the most out of practice learning. If we are stressed, if we are tired, if we are not eating correctly, we are not going to be fully present in the practice learning environment.

Complete this activity now
Thought experiment

I want you to imagine a time in your life (this can be real or imaginary) when you have been tired and hungry. Now I want you to imagine that you are on a busy ward, there are three service users all vying for your attention and your practice assessor has told you to don your personal protective equipment and come to watch them perform a new skill and demonstrate it back to them after.

- How well do you think you will be able to pick up the new skill?
- What could *you* change in this scenario to make sure you are a more effective learner?

Self-care is the corner stone of being a resilient practitioner. By self-care, I mean the whole range of actions that people do to look after themselves. This can be ranging from eating the correct food, getting a full night's sleep, to making sure that you are not over working your hours when on placement. It is important to work within the Working Time Regulations (1998) 48-hour maximum a week. When we are in a state of self-care, we are better able to care for others. Not only that, but we are also better placed to learn how to care for others. I do want to extend the notion of self-care, however, Chapter 6 of this text discusses this further. There is a tendency to see self-care as a bubble bath or buying a new pair of shoes. While these are important, we need to see the practice as much small things, to ensure they are not being missed. I argue that paying your bills on time is self-care, because they will not pile up and cause you stress at the end of the month. Doing university work in little blocks is also self-care, because then you will not have to rush at the deadline.

Write here

Use this space below to create a list of things (there is nothing too small) that you can do on placement that will be practicing self-care:

After/ending placement

With your placement at an end, you might think to yourself that there is nothing more you need to do to maximise your learning, and while technically all your learning from the area might be finished you need to be able to demonstrate that learning to your academic assessor. To do this, you need to make sure you check your PAD/ePAD is fully completed before your final interview. There can be many issues with leaving bits of your PAD/ePAD undone; for example, you may have forgotten to sign off an episode of care, which is picked up by your academic assessor. They will tell you to go back to your placement area and get this signed. On the face of things not too bad, but we know that staff move around health care settings a lot, there is sickness, and other types of leave. This means you might not be able to get your episode of care signed off. This could mean that you must repeat the episode of care at a future placement, or if this is your last placement of the part there could be bigger issues. Part of making the most out of your learning is making sure that the learning you have done can be evidenced and used to your progression and advantage.

Make sure you fill out your placement feedback. Doing this is an expression of professional kindness. A placement area is not just for yourself, but for countless other student nurses as well, as such it is important for placement areas to know what they can do to improve their student learning. That is why feedback is so important. It is also another time for you to learn, or practice, some skills. Giving feedback can be difficult, especially if you feel you have not got the most out of a placement area (for whatever reason) and taking the emotion out of a negative experience and giving feedback that will allow a placement area to grow for future students is a duty that student nurses should take seriously.

Hear It from the student

Serena's advice

My experiences of placement have been mostly pleasant. I made sure to contact my assessors beforehand by email, so that they knew who I was and to ask any questions I had. I always planned my journeys ahead of time and visited the location to ensure that I knew where I would be going. During my time on placement, I would write a list of things I was interested in learning about, skills I would want to improve on and wards/areas I'd want to have insight on. When planning my schedule, I would discuss with my practice assessor the days I could work except for Sundays, due to therapy, which they were happy to work around. To ensure I got the most out of my placements, I asked to sit in MDT meetings and contributed, attend therapy groups (with permission), visit clients and lead on interviews and assisted in writing patient notes. I worked alongside a variety of experienced healthcare professionals, with whom I learned a great deal from, these relationships really helped in adding to the placement experience.

Health and wellbeing

Making sure I had adequate sleep was very important to me, as working 12 hour shifts three to four times a week can be very tiring; especially if you are scheduled to work back-to-back shifts. I tried to space my shifts out (unless I worked in the community then I worked Monday to Friday). After a long day, soon as I got home, I would go straight to bed if I had to be in the next day. On my days off, I would sleep in, maybe go to the gym and make my lunch for the next few days. It was important for me not to overexert and check in with myself from time to time to make sure mentally, emotionally, and physically I was okay. The days that I felt uneasy, I would speak to my academic guidance tutor at the university for advice or check in with my therapist. It can be challenging at times to put yourself first while on placement as you can get so preoccupied with looking after your patient's, that your wellbeing becomes second nature, but I have learnt to prioritise myself first, so that I can show up and look after the patients to the best of my ability.

I recall a time that I had sat in on an MDT meeting with a patient, doctor and nurse and after listening to the patient's story, I left immediately to break down in tears. Thankfully, I was able to speak to one of the mental health nurses, who reassured me and reminded me that it was okay to cry, and I did the right thing not to break down in front of the patient. Again, it is very important to check in with yourself and speak to your assessor regarding any concerns you may have, to not overwhelm yourself or feel as if you are alone.

In summary, placement is an exciting place to gain valuable experience and to get a taste of what it is to work in your chosen profession. It challenges you to think as a professional healthcare worker with the added support of having an experienced team. It is important to take initiative and be enthusiastic about your work environment, it will leave a lasting impression on your colleagues and patients. As healthcare workers are priority is always the patients, but it is equally important to take care of ourselves and do what we can to ensure we are functioning at an optimum level.

Serena, student nurse mental health field

Hear it from the student
Laura's advice

I am currently a second-year student in my adult nursing training programme at and I can confidently say that over my two years of study, I have had both positive and negative placement experiences but overall, I have always been made to feel welcome and supported which made my placements great places to learn.

The following are some tips to help you with your placements and, hopefully, have a positive placement experience.

Prior to placement: make contact

Contacting clinical placements is the initial step in preparing for clinical placements. Send them an email and introduce yourself as soon as you know where your next placement will be. Clinical placements are important, but they can be terrifying if you do not know what to anticipate. Familiarise yourself with the speciality of your placement and find out what kind of clinical skills you will be using during your placement. This is necessary since you will find that some placements will not provide you with the same exposure as others. Determine your working hours as well. Working hours will vary according to the placement. Nurses in the community are more likely to work shorter day shifts than their colleagues in the hospital, who tend to work long shifts. Make your shifts as flexible as possible so that you work the same shifts as your practice assessor or practice supervisor and work alongside them whenever possible to maximise your learning possibilities.

During placement: be organised and punctual

My second top recommendation for placement is to be organised and have all the necessary nursing materials available, set dates for your interviews with your assessors/mentors in advance and set yourself goals to achieve all the learning objectives. You will be working in a professional environment, so be punctual. In any field of healthcare, handover is very important, and if you are late, you might lose important information for the patient you are providing care to. Always bring/ use a tiny notebook that fits in your pocket when on placement to log hours, take notes, make short thoughts, and so on, always adhere to the rules of confidentiality!

Ask lots of questions

The third tip is to ask a lot of questions. Asking a lot of questions shows that you are inquisitive, interested and keen to learn, which is a good impression to make. If you do not understand what is being asked of you, ask questions. If your practice assessor or practice supervisor is unavailable, consider speaking with other members of the healthcare team. Recognise when you need assistance and ask for it. Engage with everyone, from cleaners to doctors (as appropriate). They are all part of the team, and you are part of that team when on placement.

Keep on track with your clinical hours

The fourth tip I have is to keep track of your clinical hours. Knowing how many hours you have completed is easier with the new online ePAD system. Some circumstances are beyond our control and you may find yourself falling behind on hours. This may not seem important in the first year but believe me when I say that all your missed clinical hours add up. We are expected to work a certain number of hours as student nurses, and the last thing you want is to be short on hours and must extend your placement when everyone is graduating.

Never miss a learning opportunity

My fifth tip for nursing placement recommendation is to never pass up an opportunity to learn. As a student nurse, you have the best opportunity to learn. When you have your initial meeting with your practice assessor or supervisor and outline the goals you want to achieve in your placement. You should definitely consider expanding beyond the area of the placement that you are allocated. Be proactive and explore all of the fantastic outreach options that are available that can benefit your practice! Be sure to research up on the new things you are learning on placement and do not be shy about asking to sort out the medication trolley. This will help you with your pharmacology and medicine management.

Look after your health

My second-to-last piece of advice for preparing for placements is to prioritise your health and well-being as a student nurse during clinical placements, and to use your free days to recharge your batteries when you're not working and do the things you love to do. Do not take things too personally. Especially from patients as they probably do not mean it and your probably not the problem at all but just so happen to be in the firing line. However, if it is particularly inappropriate then it must be shared with your assessor or reported.

On completion of placement: reflection

Last, but not least, remember to reflect both during and after placement; it will help your personal development by increasing self-awareness. Reflection is also important in improving patient care since it aids in the expansion and development of clinical knowledge and abilities. Always uphold our Code of Conduct and the '6 Cs of nursing', which are the key principles and expectations drawn from the profession, including altruism, autonomy, human dignity, integrity, honesty, and social justice.

PS Do not forget to wear comfortable shoes and compression stockings for those long shifts!!! And take pack lunch and save those pennies!!!

Laura, student nurse adult field

Summary

Placement learning is the time when you, as a student nurse, can practice your skills, embed your learning and develop into a nurse. It is filled with challenges and rewards, emotions, and most importantly learning. If you take on board what you are taught at university and what you have read in this chapter (as well as the other chapters in this book) you will maximise your own learning on placement and become the best nurse you can be. There are lots of things to bear in mind when on placement, so much so that it can feel overwhelming. It can be simplified into three sentences of advice: know the area you are going to, be eager to learn, and reflect on what you have learnt. I wish you all the best in your journey in becoming a nurse.

References

Gibbs, G. (1988). *Learning by Doing: A Guide to Teaching and Learning Methods*. Oxford: Oxford Polytechnic.

Health Education England (2021). *Importance of Reflection in Good Competency Evidence*. https://nshcs.hee.nhs.uk/services/train-the-trainer/stp-train-the-trainer/guide-to-producing-good-competency-evidence/the-importance-of-reflection-in-good-competency-evidence (accessed 15 August 2022).

Nursing and Midwifery Council (2018). *Realising Professionalism: Standards for Education and Training. Part 2: Standards for Student Supervision and Assessment*. www.nmc.org.uk/student-supervision-assessment (accessed 15 August 2022).

Schön, D. (1983). *The Reflective Practitioner: How Professionals Think in Action*. New York, NY: Basic Books.

Taylor, B. (2010). *Reflective Practice for Healthcare Professionals*. London: McGraw-Hill.

Walsh, M. and Ford, P. (1989). *Nursing Rituals, Research and Rational Actions*. London: Butterworth-Heinemann.

Standards for student supervision and assessment

Jo Rixon

AIM

This chapter presents the reader with an overview of the Nursing and Midwifery Council (NMC) Standards for Student Supervision and Assessment (SSSA).

LEARNING OUTCOMES

Having read this chapter, the reader will:

1. Demonstrate an awareness of the NMC SSSA.
2. Be aware of the roles identified by the NMC responsible for support, supervision and assessment.
3. Describe the specific responsibility for each of the identified roles and how they support learning.
4. Understand how students are assessed for theory and practice.

Succeeding on your Nursing Placement: Supervision, Learning and Assessment for Nursing Students, First Edition. Edited by Ian Peate.
© 2024 John Wiley & Sons Ltd. Published 2024 by John Wiley & Sons Ltd.

Introduction

In Chapter 2, the suite of standards established by the NMC in 2018 was introduced. One part of this suite of standards is the SSSA (NMC 2018a). This standard outlines the NMC's expectations as to how all students on an NMC approved course would be supported with their learning and supervised in clinical practice, and how they would be assessed for theory and practice.

When considering practice learning for pre-registration students, it is also important to consider the NMC requirements within both the Part 1 standards framework for nursing and midwifery education (NMC 2018b) and the programme-specific standards for pre-registration nursing and the nursing associate (NMC 2018c, 2018d). These standards set out requirements relating to the quality of programme provision and the skills and knowledge required for entry to the professional register. This chapter explores specifically the SSSA (NMC 2018a). It outlines the different roles and the responsibilities for each of these roles in supporting the learning, supervision, and assessment of students to facilitate progression and assurance of student achievement and competence.

An overview of the standards

While individual universities and programmes will arrange the student's practice placements differently, the NMC has set standards to ensure that supervision and assessment is fair and consistent. This chapter explores the guidance set out by the NMC to ensure that students are supervised and assessed appropriately within practice placements.

In May 2018, the NMC released a new suite of standards to support pre-registration nursing, nursing associate and midwifery students to achieve the required proficiencies and programme standards to enter the NMC register (NMC 2018c, 2018d, 2018e). Included in this suite is the Part 2: SSSA (NMC 2018a) which replaced the Standards for Learning and Assessment in Practice (SLAiP) (NMC 2008). Initially, universities and practice learning partners were expected to take a considered approach to transition onto the new standards as staff developed into the new roles. With the impact of COVID-19, the introduction was expedited with all universities and practice learning partners required to implement the standards in May 2020 under the NMC Emergency Standards (NMC 2020).

Previously, SLAiP (NMC 2008) had required nursing and midwifery students to spend a minimum of 40% of their time while in clinical practice under the direct supervision of their assigned mentor, who would be responsible for the completion of the summative assessment of the student's practice learning. The mentor was someone who had undertaken formal training and was 'qualified' as a mentor, as described by SLAiP (NMC 2008). In addition, on completion of the final placement, students were required to be 'signed off' by their allocated 'sign-off mentor'. The sign-off mentor was an experienced mentor who had undertaken additional training and was appointed to make the final decision on whether the nursing or midwifery student had met all the clinical practice requirements of the programme, was fit for practice and therefore could be recommended for admission to the NMC register. Box 8.1 provides a summary of the key differences between the two sets of standards.

Box 8.1 | Summary of key differences between the Standards for Student Supervision and Assessment and the Standards for Learning and Assessment in Practice

- The term mentor is no longer used.
- Triennial review no longer required.
- New roles of practice assessor, practice supervisor, nominated person and academic assessor have been introduced.
- Specific university level preparation not required for practice assessor and practice supervisor role.
- All registered nurses are responsible for contributing to the supervision and support of students in practice.
- Any registered healthcare professional can act as supervisors for students.
- Practice supervisors will support students in practice providing feedback to practice assessors to inform decision making.
- Practice assessors and academic assessors to collaborate.
- Students are no longer required to spend a designated percentage of their placement time with a specific practice supervisor of practice assessor. Previously, students spent 40% of their time working under the direct supervision of the mentor.

Source: NMC (2008, 2018a).

Complete this activity now

- Consider what the term 'mentor' means to you.

- Have you had an identified mentor before? What was their role?

The new standards have three fundamental ambitions. First, supporting students to feel empowered and able to take responsibility for their own learning, planning with their supervisor the clinical experiences required to achieve their proficiencies. Linked with this was the NMC's desire to reduce the risk of 'failure to fail', as previously explored by Duffy (2003). Previously, the mentor was supervisor and assessor; however now the roles are segregated to make the process more robust and objective. In addition, the NMC wanted to increase flexibility in relation to practice learning, encouraging universities and practice learning partners to be innovative in their approaches to nursing and midwifery education. The SSSA outlines the NMC's expectations and the processes required to ensure that nursing, nursing associate and midwifery students are provided with an appropriate learning environment, as well as how they will be supported, supervised and assessed in the practice environment. The NMC recognises that everyone can play a part in the learning experience of the student, registered and non-registered staff, including other students. A feature here is the emphasis on the NMC requirement, as articulated in the Code (NMC 2018f), for all registrants (nurses, midwives, and nursing associates) to support the learning of others: 'support students' and colleagues' learning to help them develop their professional competence and confidence' (NMC 2018f, 9.4)

As well as now identifying the supervision of students as everyone's responsibility, the removal of the requirements attached to the mentor role allows for increased flexibility in approaches to the supervision of students. Assessment of learning is also a fundamental aspect of the process, and therefore within the standards. The NMC outlines its expectations of how students should be assessed in both theory and practice. To articulate these requirements clearly to all, the NMC has presented them under three headings (Table 8.1).

TABLE 8.1

Sections of the Standard for Student Supervision and Assessment.

Section	Description
Effective practice learning (1)	These standards describe what needs to be in place to deliver safe and effective learning experiences for nursing and midwifery students in practice.
Supervision of students (2–5)	These standards describe the principles of student supervision in the practice environment and the role of the practice supervisor.
Assessment of students and confirmation of proficiency (6–10)	These standards set out what is required from educators who are assessing and confirming students' practice and academic achievement. They describe the role and responsibilities of the practice and academic assessor

Source: Adapted from NMC (2018a).

There are many people who will support the student. As already identified, the NMC no longer requires mentors; however, they have identified three new roles to support the supervision and assessment of nursing, nursing associate and midwifery students. The three roles are:

- practice supervisor
- practice assessor
- academic assessor.

The rest of this chapter explores the NMC's requirements for practice learning support, supervision and student assessment, together with an explanation of the three new associated roles.

Go online

Access these resources, which have been made available by the NMC:

Standards for student supervision and assessment: www.nmc.org.uk/standards-for-education-and-training/standards-for-student-supervision-and-assessment

Supporting information on standards for student supervision and assessment: www.nmc.org.uk/supporting-information-on-standards-for-student-supervision-and-assessment

Learning environments (organisation of practice learning)

In developing the new standards, the NMC aimed to allow for local innovation in programme delivery but also set clear standards to ensure that nursing, nursing associate and midwifery students receive safe, effective and inclusive learning experiences. In addition, they aimed to support students to actively participate in their own learning experience, encouraging students to learn from a broad range of people while completing practice placements in a wide variety of settings.

To guide universities and practice learning partners in the provision of effective learning, the NMC has provided a number of standards that describe what needs to be in place to ensure the 'organisation of practice learning' (NMC 2018a). The NMC identifies the need for there to be suitable systems, processes, resources and individuals in place to facilitate safe and effective learning. Responding to this and the continuing challenge of meeting the demand for sufficient quality practice placements, in 2021, Health Education England (HEE) (HEE 2021) provided practice placement providers the opportunity to access funding to support the expansion of placement opportunities. This funding was to support innovative projects but a proviso of the funding was that the projects still needed to comply with NMC and programme standards and support students to meet the proficiencies relevant to their programme. The prerequisites set by HEE fit with the initial standard set by the NMC for practice learning. The NMC standards relate to the need for practice learning to comply with the NMC standards framework for nursing and midwifery education (NMC 2018b) and programme specific standards, as well as support achievement of proficiencies and relevant programme outcomes.

Students need to achieve their learning outcomes through the provision of safe and effective learning opportunities. Those opportunities not only need to be safe for the student but also for patients and the public. To ensure the safety of patients and the public, students need to practise within their capability and be supervised while developing their proficiency. To ensure provision of quality learning opportunities in safe learning environments, universities need assurance from the placement providers that the NMC standards and regulatory requirements are adhered to. This is often achieved through the completion of a practice learning environment audit and should be available for students to review. A key element considered within the audit is resources, both in relation to the learning opportunities available and the staff available to provide supervision and support for learning.

In relation to staff resources, an additional role identified is the 'nominated person'. This is a separate role to the three main roles identified for supporting supervision and assessment in practice placements. This role is identified as a person who must be available to support the students and be familiar with university and placement provider processes for managing concerns. They may not necessarily be based within the learning environment but should be able to support students who escalate concerns.

> ## Complete this activity now
>
> Consider what the NMC states is your role in relation to maintaining patient/service user/public safety. What is your university process for escalating concerns?

The NMC does not set out how many staff are needed to support students or who should do what in relation to organising the practice learning experience. As already detailed, it does identify three specific roles within the standards to support learning: practice supervisor, practice assessor and academic assessor. The NMC also describes where it is acceptable for students to be in areas that offer the opportunity to not be directly supervised by their identified practice supervisor/s or practice assessor but where a suitable person has oversight of their learning. This would apply in such instances when enrichment or spoke opportunities exist, where there may be no registered health or social care professional available (Figure 8.1). The person coordinating the activity would need to ensure that the student and the person supporting the student's learning have a clear understanding of learning outcomes to be achieved and the support required.

Students are required to gain experience across a range of different learning environments in a range of care situations to meet the programme learning outcomes. These could include a variety of health and social care settings such as a mix of hospital, community and independent environments. The practice learning environment auditing process will assist in identifying the learning experiences available within each of the environments, including opportunities to engage in spoke activities, follow pathways of care or interprofessional learning activities.

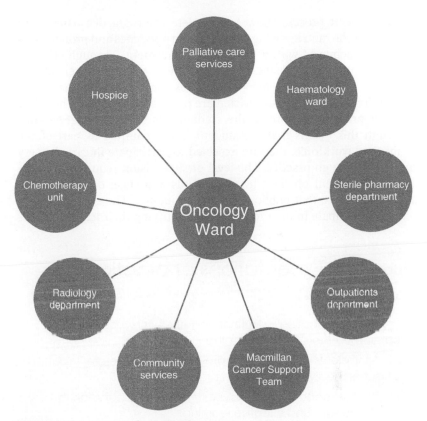

FIGURE 8.1 The concept of a spoke placement.

Over to you

Consider what the clinical placement area you going to next can offer as spoke and interprofessional learning opportunities.

Practice supervision and the role of the student

The student has a key role to play in ensuring that they achieve the learning required for their programme. It is essential that the student takes responsibility for their own learning by both understanding the assessment process (how to complete their practice assessment documentation) and knowing what learning outcomes and proficiencies need to be achieved within the practice placement. Through effective practice supervision and student empowerment, students are enabled to learn and safely achieve the proficiencies for their programme. The expectations of practice supervision are outlined in Box 8.2.When they are in a practice placement, the student has supernumerary status. Although this means that the student is not counted as part of the established workforce, they are expected to participate in care delivery and learn through practice. The level of supervision required by a student is dependent on their learning needs and stage of learning but must also ensure that public safety is maintained. The student should actively participate in their learning by identifying their learning needs

---

Box 8.2 | Expectations of practice supervision

Approved education institutions, together with practice learning partners, must ensure that:

2.1 All students on an NMC approved programme are supervised while learning in practice.

2.2 There is support and oversight of practice supervision to ensure safe and effective learning.

2.3 The level of supervision provided to students reflects their learning needs and stage of learning.

2.4 Practice supervision ensures safe and effective learning experiences that uphold public protection and the safety of people.

2.5 There is sufficient coordination and continuity of support and supervision of students to ensure safe and effective learning experiences.

2.6 Practice supervision facilitates independent learning.

2.7 All students on an NMC approved programme are supervised in practice by NMC registered nurses, midwives, nursing associates and other registered health and social care professionals.

Source: Adapted from NMC (2018a).

in advance of the clinical placement, by actively seeking out learning opportunities to achieve the NMC proficiencies and reflect on the learning achieved.

> **Over to you**
>
> As a student, you should seek feedback from staff, service users and peers on your performance. When you receive this feedback, reflect on it using a recognised model of reflection and consider ways in which this feedback can support your learning.

Practice supervisor's roles and responsibilities

The aim of practice supervision is to enable students to learn and safely achieve their required proficiencies. Within the SSSA (NMC 2018a), the NMC identifies that all students must be supervised by an assigned practice supervisor while learning in practice. A student may have more than one assigned supervisor. Those taking on the role must be appropriately prepared for the role and receive continuing support to fulfil the role (preparation is covered later in the chapter). Practice supervisors can be:

- registered nurses
- midwives
- nursing associates
- paramedics
- pharmacists
- any registered health and social care professional.

Practice supervisors are identified to take on the role and are required to act as role models, in line with their relevant codes of conduct.

How the practice supervisor provides the supervision may vary depending on the environment and the learning to be achieved. The practice supervisor would also be aware of the need to consider any equality and diversity needs, working with a student to make appropriate reasonable adjustments as identified for the student. As already identified, non-registered health and social care providers can play a part in supporting student learning. This is a significant change from the previous standards where students were required to spend at least 40% of their time allocated in the practice placement, working the same shift, under the supervision of their mentor. With the increased flexibility afforded by the new standards, with the practice supervisor maintaining a degree of oversight, others may be called upon to support the learning experience depending on:

- the skill being taught
- the experience of the person
- the environment.

Examples of where this may be used could be phlebotomists, teachers, custody staff or social prescribers.

Hear it from the student

'While on my placement at a general practice, I spent some time with the receptionist. This was a really useful experience to help me understand some of the challenges associated with managing the booking system and co-ordinating the home visits for the GPs. The main skill I saw in practice though was communication. They had to communicate in so many different ways, showing empathy to those who were unwell or upset and de-escalating conflict with those who were unhappy when appointments were running late or when they couldn't get an appointment when they wanted it.'

Elisha, first-year learning disabilities student nurse

This first-year student comment demonstrates how learning can come from many sources and not just from the practice supervisor or the practice assessor. It therefore highlights the importance of a student considering other sources of learning while in a practice placement. When the practice supervisor is considering learning opportunities for the student, they will ensure the student is not placed in a situation that is outside of the student capability. At this point, it is also important that a student acknowledges and shares their limitations and learning needs. Sharing with the practice supervisor will enable them to draw on their experience and knowledge to judge what may be appropriate for the student and the environment. They will then be able to provide or arrange tailored learning opportunities to meet the student learning needs, to support achievement of proficiencies and skills.

Students are encouraged to consider and prepare for a discussion with the practice supervisor about their learning needs, which will take place at the commencement of their practice placement. The practice supervisor will then work with the student to turn the learning needs into learning objectives, prioritising the learning needs and planning suitable learning opportunities to meet the identified objectives. The important feature of the practice supervisor role is to support the process of learning by developing a professional relationship with the student, where the student looks at the practice supervisor as a role model and is comfortable to ask questions that will support growth and development.

Practice learning is a continuous process, and is a crucial component of the process is the provision of feedback. The giving of feedback may have one of three purposes:

1. Constructive, supplying feedback on overall general performance.
2. Specific, advising on progress in relation to conduct and professional behaviour or achievement of skills and proficiencies.
3. Developing an action plan to support performance.

Feedback should focus on the present and the future, allowing the practice supervisor and the student to discuss experiences, share ideas and explore ways of moving forward together. Students should not see the receiving of feedback as a critical or negative experience but as opportunity to reflect and develop with the supervision and coaching of an appropriately experienced nurse, midwife, nursing associate or health and social care professional.

The giving and recording of feedback is covered in detail in Chapters 9 and 10, but it is important to acknowledge here that although feedback may be given orally, it is also important that feedback from both the practice supervisor and others who support learning for the student is recorded in the student's practice assessment document. This record of conduct, proficiency and achievement supports the practice assessor in their assessment of the student performance.

Write here

How do you respond to feedback, do you prefer this be oral or written? Write down key points regarding feedback (refer also to Chapters 9 and 10 of this text).

Practice supervisors: contribution to assessment and progression

During a practice placement, the student will have numerous opportunities to learn and develop their skills and to demonstrate their growth in confidence and competence. It is unlikely that all opportunities to demonstrate this professional development will be witnessed by a practice assessor. It is for this reason that the practice supervisor plays a key role in supporting the assessment process and playing a part in ensuring informed decisions for progression.

Over to you

- Thinking about your last placement, what specific activities did you engage in that your practice supervisor specifically documented to ensure your practice assessor was aware of your performance?

- Were there any activities you did not document that now, on reflection, may have been useful so you could explore these experiences with your practice assessor to evidence your development and competence?

- If this going to be your first placement, try to contact a student who has already been on placement and discuss these issues with them. Review your discussion after your placement and make a comparison.

While supervising the student, if the practice supervisor becomes concerned about the students conduct or competence, they should raise this concern with the practice assessor and academic assessor. Failure to meet the requirements of a practice placement may result in the student being referred within that practice placement area; this may have implications for the student's progression, depending on specific programme requirements. If a concern is raised, all parties should work in a supportive and collaborative way to address the concerns and facilitate improvement in the student's performance. This may result in an action plan being implemented to ensure the student is aware of what needs to be achieved and to enable to practice supervisor to direct their support and supervision towards achieving the required outcomes. Box 8.3 gives some tips for raising concerns as a student.

Box 8.3 | How to raise concerns

If you need to raise concerns about any aspects of your learning experience most universities have protocols in place. It is essential to remember that raising a concern about your learning experience is different to escalating a concern in relation to patient/service user/public safety as considered earlier.

A general approach to seeking support with your practice learning experience is to approach those closest to the situation who may be able to help. In the first instance consider speaking to practice supervisor or practice assessor about your learning needs and the support you need to achieve these. Additional people to approach within the practice environment would be the department or ward manager/sister/charge nurse or the person identified as the nominated person for student support

Your university will also have support structures in place, people you can approach such as link lecturer's who visit you in placement, your academic assessor or your personal tutor.

Your learning is your responsibility so it is important you follow the correct channel to get support should you need it.

Throughout the practice placement the practice supervisor will take opportunities to engage with the practice assessor and academic assessor to share information on relevant observations and the progression of the student. In addition, a fundamental route for sharing this information is via the student's practice assessment documentation (see Chapter 9). It is for this reason that it is essential that the student makes their practice assessment documentation available to the practice supervisor, whether this be a hard copy document or electronic document. The practice supervisor should be making regular entries and recording the student's achievements, including relevant observations of their conduct and proficiency for the practice assessor to review.

The practice supervisor has an important role to play in supporting learning and assessment, which requires knowledge and skills to conduct the role effectively. By showing a willingness to share their knowledge and skills, the student will feel confident that the practice supervisor has the competence to support their learning. It is also important that the practice assessor is confident in the feedback the practice supervisor is sharing with them. This therefore reinforces the importance of preparation for the role and ongoing support.

Assessor's roles

The standards require assessment and confirmation of proficiency to be based on the student's achievement across theory and practice. To provide assurance of the student achievement and competence, the assessments need to be evidence based, robust and objective. To support this process, the NMC (2018a) has introduced two roles associated with assessment: practice assessor and academic assessor.

To support the validity of these assessments, all assessor roles are required to be either registered nurses or nursing associates. Those taking on the role must be appropriately prepared and receive continuing support to fulfil the role (preparation is covered later in the chapter). A specific requirement to assure the legitimacy of the assessment for nursing students is that the practice assessor and academic assessor have appropriate equivalent experience for the student's field of practice.

Green flag

Assessor experience requirements are different for midwives, specialist community public health nurses and post-registration courses.

As well as confirming proficiency, the practice assessor and academic assessor need to be prepared to raise and respond to concerns. These concerns may relate to student conduct, competence or achievement, and may be identified by either of the assigned assessors or by one of the assigned practice supervisors. To assist in situations where a concern has been raised, universities and practice learning partners should have appropriate processes and support in place for the practice and academic assessor. In some circumstances, the nominated person may also become involved at this point.

With regard to assignment, the practice assessor and academic assessor need to meet the criteria as outlined above, including having undergone appropriate preparation for the role. The student should be assigned an identified practice assessor per episode of practice assessment, which may equate to a practice placement or a series of practice placements, depending on the programme structure. While a student may be assigned a number of practice supervisors at any one time, they should only have the one practice assessor per episode of assessment. A student should also only be assigned one academic assessor at a time and must be allocated a different person as academic assessor for each part of the education programme.

An additional role assignment requirement is that no person is undertaking more than one of the identified roles for an individual student (i.e. the practice supervisor cannot be the practice assessor for the same student); however, they could be practice assessor for one student and practice supervisor for an alternative student. The NMC implemented the requirement for separate people to undertake the roles to increase the robustness in the decision making and assessment process, removing the responsibility from just one person, as was the case with mentors. See Table 8.2 for a summary of the criteria for role assignment.

TABLE 8.2

Criteria for role assignment.

Role	Criteria
Practice supervisor	Must be a nurse, nursing associate or any registered health and social care professional. Must have had suitable preparation for role. Can have more than one practice supervisor. Cannot also be practice assessor or academic assessor.
Practice assessor	Must be a nurse or nursing associate. (For nursing students must have experience within same field as student). Must have suitable preparation for role. Assigned for a specific placement or series of placements. Cannot also be practice supervisor or academic assessor.
Academic assessor	Must be a nurse or nursing associate (for nursing students must have experience within same field as student). Must have suitable preparation for role. Different academic assessor to be assigned per part of the programme. Cannot also be practice supervisor or practice assessor.

Source: Adapted from NMC (2018a).

Practice assessor responsibilities

The practice assessor is assigned per episode of practice assessment. The assigned practice assessor should have relevant knowledge and/or experience of working within the clinical placement area itself or within the specialism to assess and confirm the proficiencies and programme outcomes. It is not a requirement that the practice assessor is physically based or employed within the area of practice, but they must be able to gather sufficient information to make an evidence based, objective assessment of the student's achievement of proficiencies and practice learning related programme outcomes.

To conduct an assessment, the practice assessor needs to collate information and feedback from a number of sources. This gathering and coordinating feedback from the assigned practice supervisor/s and others is key in facilitating the decision-making process. For this reason, it is important that the student gathers regular feedback from a variety of sources and takes the opportunity to record and reflect on learning opportunities within the practice assessment documentation for the practice assessor to refer to. The practice assessor should also have an insight into the student's history, not only of their progress within practice but also their progress within theory component of the programme. In addition, as identified with the practice supervisor, it is also important for the student to share with the practice assessor any particular reasonable adjustments that may need to be taken into consideration when conducting assessments.

Over to you

- Thinking about your last placement, what evidence did you collect to support your practice assessor in making their decision? What additional evidence do you think you could collect next time?

- If you are preparing for your first placement, think about what you might be able to collect. Review this after your placement to see if you gathered any evidence, you hadn't thought of before the placement.

Assessment should be a continuous process, where reviewing the feedback from others should be undertaken periodically during the assessment period and not just at the end. A continuous review of the feedback being collated will ensure that the practice assessor has sufficient evidence to make a fair and objective assessment of the student. In addition to seeking feedback from others, the practice assessor will periodically take opportunities to observe the student in the practice placement. This may be observing from a distance while the student works with the practice supervisor, working directly with the student or undertaking a summative aspect of assessment depending on the education programme requirements (e.g. the practice assessor may be required to conduct a summative assessment of the student's medicines management skills and therefore administer medicines with them). When making the assessment of the student's conduct, proficiency and achievement the practice assessor will provide the student with oral feedback on progress as well as recording the assessments within the student's practice assessment document.

Green flag

Where possible and if appropriate, you are encouraged to seek out opportunities to work with other members of the multidisciplinary team. Doing this can enhance your knowledge and understanding of the various roles in the health and care professions.

If a practice assessor becomes concerned regarding a student's performance or a concern is raised by the practice supervisor, the practice assessor must then take a role in improving the student's performance. This may result in the need for an action plan to be developed and implemented by the practice supervisor or the practice assessor to work more directly with the student. Any action would normally be a joint decision involving the practice assessor, practice supervisor, academic assessor and the student. If it becomes apparent that the student is not going to achieve the requirements of the educational programme for that practice learning episode, the practice assessor should take appropriate action. The action to be taken may be recommending the practice placement be failed and/ or the student should not be recommended for progression. This would be managed in collaboration with the academic assessor to ensure the necessary university processes are followed.

Throughout the episode of practice, the practice assessor and academic assessor should work in partnership, regularly communicating and collaborating to review the student's progress. At the point of progression, the practice assessor should also consider if the student demonstrates the conduct and professional values required of the professional role. Both assessors should bring their expertise and scope of practice to the process to support the final decision for progression.

Academic assessor responsibilities

The academic assessor is a new concept introduced by the SSSA (NMC 2018a). An academic assessor is assigned per part of the educational programme and should have relevant knowledge and experience to assess and confirm the proficiencies and programme outcomes in the academic environment.

In summary, the role of the academic assessor is similar to that of the practice assessor, focusing primarily on the academic work of the student. The academic assessor is responsible for collating, confirming and documenting an evidence-based objective assessment of the student's academic performance. They should be working to support the student's academic performance, reviewing academic progress and providing regular feedback for the student. Sources of evidence to support the academic assessor's decision may include academic work assessment outcomes, communications from academic staff and communication from the student.

The practice assessor and the academic assessor should be working in partnership, regularly communicating and collaborating to review student progress. Should a concern be raised in regard to the student's performance in the practice placement, the academic assessor would work in collaboration with the practice supervisor and practice assessor to support improvement in the student's performance.

At the point of progression, the recommendation for progression should be a shared process between the two assessors, confirming that the student has achieved the proficiencies and learning outcomes of the education programme for progressions, as well as demonstrating the conduct and professional values of the professional role.

Role preparation

Whilst the NMC no longer mandates specific training requirements as they did with mentorship and SLAiP (NMC 2008), it does identify specific standards relating to preparation for the three identified roles. One of the standards is clearly the need to understand the proficiencies and programme outcomes required for the student they are supporting (NMC 2018a); being able to support learning, give feedback and conduct assessments is reliant on knowing what needs to be achieved. Different approaches may be taken by universities to share this information with practice supervisors, practice assessors and academic assessors. This may be via briefing sessions, online learning resources or hard documents. A valuable source of this information is also the student, who should be aware of their programme requirements and the practice assessment document that should give guidance on assessment requirements and completion of the document.

A practice supervisor's notes

When a student arrives for their placement, it is really helpful if they come prepared. It is so difficult to support the students learning if they have no idea what they want and, more importantly, what they need to achieve during the placement to meet their programme requirements. The student is the best person to identify their strengths and limitations and therefore where their focus needs to be so I can then provide the learning opportunities to meet the programme requirements.

Depending on the previous experience and professional qualification of the person undertaking a role and the actual role to be undertaken, the preparation will vary. The key focus of any preparation is to ensure that the person supporting student learning feels adequately prepared and is supported to reflect and continue to develop the skills required in their role. Having confident and competent practice supervisors and practice assessors within a practice placement should instil a positive learning culture and, therefore, a positive learning opportunity for the student.

To address the different responsibilities of the roles, the NMC has identified preparation and learning required to prepare for the roles. The practice supervisor is required to have skills in effective supervision and the ability to contribute to student learning and assessment. The practice assessor and academic assessor require additional skills, the focus of which is interpersonal communication skills and the ability to give constructive feedback. In addition, as their role focuses on the assessment of the student, they require knowledge of the assessment process and their role within it, and the knowledge and skills required to conduct objective, evidence-based assessments (NMC 2018a).

The preparation and continuing support required is at the discretion of the university and the practice learning partner and will also be dependent on the experience and professional background of the person taking on the role. For nursing and nursing associate students registering against the NMC 2018 standards, their programmes of study include practice supervisor preparation (NMC 2018c, 2018d). Therefore, at the point of qualifying, these registrants will be prepared to take on the role of practice supervisor. In many organisations, registered nurses who have previously undertaken NMC approved mentorship training, would be transitioned directly to the role of practice assessor following familiarisation with the new standards and programme requirements. For those nurses who have never completed mentorship training (registered pre-2018 standards), nursing associates (registered pre-2018 standards) or other registered health and social care professionals, different requirements of study may be required. An example of the preparation that may be implemented is shown in Table 8.3.

There may be additional people involved in facilitating and providing learning opportunities with the practice placement, and their feedback to the practice supervisor and practice assessor is valid. It is, however, the practice supervisor's responsibility when coordinating such activities to ensure the activity is acceptable with the university and that the person

---

TABLE 8.3

Example of preparation for those with no previous experience of supporting student learning in practice.

Practice supervisor	Practice assessor
Familiarisation with proficiencies and programme outcomes	Familiarisation with proficiencies and programme outcomes
Half day workshop to develop supervisory skills appropriate to supporting students in practice: • Roles and responsibilities • Assessing learning needs • Assessing learning in practice • Giving feedback • Coaching basics Additional e-learning activity: • Understanding students • Raising concerns	Full day workshop following completion of e-learning modules to develop supervisory, feedback, and assessment skills appropriate to supporting and assessing students in practice: • Roles and responsibilities • Assessing learning needs • Assessing learning in practice • Giving feedback • Coaching basics • Understanding students • Raising concerns

Source: Adapted from Pan London Practice Learning Group (2019).

facilitating the learning opportunity is aware of the student's expected learning outcomes and capabilities.

The role of the academic assessor requires the same level of knowledge and skill as the practice assessor. The preparation process for this role will be dependent on the requirements of the individual universities and on how the university implements the role.

In addition to initial preparation all those undertaking the various roles need to be given continuing support and training to develop in their roles so they can support students to be confident and competent practitioners. Despite this flexibility in provision, students can be reassured that the universities are responsible for ensuring the quality of the learning environment and the learning experience students receive.

Summary

As part of the new suite of standards from the NMC, the SSSA (NMC 2018a) were established to replace SLAiP (NMC 2008). Three new roles were established, the practice supervisor and practice assessor to replace the mentor and a new role, the academic assessor. The aim of the standards and the new roles is to ensure an effective learning experience with fairness and consistency in supervision and assessment for students. This chapter has provided an overview of the new roles and their responsibilities. It has demonstrated how the quality of the learning experience can be achieved by considering the preparation requirements for people taking on the roles of supervising and assessing students. Opportunities have also been taken within the chapter to consider the student's role, working in partnership, particularly with the practice supervisor and practice assessor, to achieve an effective learning experience which will lead to a positive practice placement outcome.

References

Duffy, K. (2003). *Failing students: a qualitative study of factors that influence the decisions regarding assessment of students' competence in practice.* https://www.researchgate.net/publication/251693467_Failing_Students_A_Qualitative_Study_of_Factors_that_Influence_the_Decisions_Regarding_Assessment_of_Students%27_Competence_in_Practice (accessed 9 July 2022).

Health Education England (2021). *Expansion of clinical placements gets a £15m boost from HEE.* http://www.hee.nhs.uk/news-blogs-events/news/expansion-clinical-placements-gets-%C2%A315m-boost-hee (accessed 9 July 2022).

Nursing and Midwifery Council (2008). *Standards to support learning and assessment in practice. NMC standards for mentors, practice teachers and teachers.* London: NMC. www.nmc.org.uk/standards-for-education-and-training/standards-to-support-learning-and-assessment-in-practice (accessed 9 July 2022).

Nursing and Midwifery Council (2018a). *Realising Professionalism: Standards for Education and Training. Part 2: Standards for Student Supervision and Assessment.* www.nmc.org.uk/Student-supervision-assessment (accessed 17 March 2023).

Nursing and Midwifery Council (2018b). *Realising Professionalism: Standards for Education and Training. Part 1: Standards Framework for Nursing and Midwifery Education.* www.nmc.org.uk/standards-for-education-and-training/standards-framework-for-nursing-and-midwifery-education (accessed 17 March 2023).

Nursing and Midwifery Council (2018c). *Realising Professionalism: Standards for Education and Training. Part 3: Standards for Pre-Registration Nursing Programmes.* www.nmc.org.uk/standards-for-education-and-training/standards-framework-for-nursing-and-midwifery-education (accessed 17 March 2023).

Nursing and Midwifery Council (2018d). *Realising Professionalism: Standards for Education and Training. Standards for Pre-Registration Nursing Associate Programmes.* www.nmc.org.uk/standards-for-education-and-training/standards-framework-for-nursing-and-midwifery-education (accessed 17 March 2023).

Nursing and Midwifery Council (2018e). *Future Nurse: Standards of Proficiency for Registered Nurses.* www.nmc.org.uk/globalassets/sitedocuments/education-standards/future-nurse-proficiencies.pdf (accessed 17 March 2023).

Nursing and Midwifery Council (2018f). *The Code. Professional standards of practice and behaviour for nurses, midwives and nursing associates.* www.nmc.org.uk/standards/code (accessed 20 July 2022)

Nursing and Midwifery Council (2020). *Emergency Standards for Nursing and Midwifery Education.* London: Nursing and Midwifery Council.

Pan London Practice Learning Group (2019). *Development Route Map.* https://plplg.uk/wp-content/uploads/2019/06/Development-Route-Map.pdf (accessed 20 July 2022).

CHAPTER 9

The practice assessment document

Jane Fish and Kathy Wilson

AIM

The aim of the chapter is to enable readers to understand the components of their practice assessment document (PAD) to support and enhance their learning and assessment in practice.

LEARNING OUTCOMES

Having read this chapter, the reader will:

1. Understand the purposes of assessment in practice, in line with Nursing and Midwifery Council (NMC) requirements.
2. Be able to identify the components of the PAD.
3. Appreciate the link between learning and assessment in practice.
4. Discuss the importance of feedback as part of the assessment process.
5. Understand how the components of the PAD help the student to achieve accountability in line with the NMC Code of Conduct (NMC 2018d) and Future Nurse Standards of proficiency for registered nurses (NMC 2018a).

Succeeding on your Nursing Placement: Supervision, Learning and Assessment for Nursing Students, First Edition. Edited by Ian Peate.
© 2024 John Wiley & Sons Ltd. Published 2024 by John Wiley & Sons Ltd.

Practice assessment documents

Students who undertake a nursing programme leading to registration must complete 2300 hours of practice hours over the course of the programme. The PAD detailed in this chapter is based on the Pan London PAD and is similar to PADs that have been adapted by many universities across England. All Wales, North Yorkshire and Humber and Manchester were among the first regions to develop a unified PAD. In 2008, NHS Scotland considered it timely to develop a national approach to student practice assessment documentation (Lauder et al. 2008). Further work led to Scotland developing a national approach where key components of the PAD were agreed across Scotland (NHS Education for Scotland 2011). In 2013, London developed their first unified PAD working with nine universities informed by the work on unified practice assessment documents across England and Wales. The evaluation of the first Pan London PAD confirmed that a unified PAD has enhanced the consistency and standardisation of student nurses' practice assessment across London (Baillie and Fish 2021).

Guidance on using the practice assessment document

The PAD is designed to support and guide students towards successfully achieving the criteria set out in Future Nurse: Standards of Proficiency for Registered Nurses (NMC 2018a) and Realising Professionalism: Standards for Education and Training Part 2 (NMC 2018b). The PAD comprises three parts and incorporates the range of Future Nurse: Standards of Proficiency (NMC 2018a). 'Parts' in this context is used to represent the range of outcomes to be achieved by students at different levels. These parts may differ from the parts of the education programme that will be defined locally by each university provider. For example, in a bachelor of science programme the parts usually align with the three academic years; however, in a two-year programme, for example masters and postgraduate diploma programmes, the definition of 'part' varies in line with local curriculum plans.

Students are required to complete each part of the PAD before they progress to the next part and, with each part, the complexity of the outcomes the student is required to achieve increases. Table 9.1 gives an example of how a two- and three-year programme within a higher education institution manages the progression points.

TABLE 9.1

Example to illustrate parts with progression points of pre-registration nursing programme.

(Progression points will vary for each university in line with their local policy)

3-yr BSc Programme		2-yr PG Dip Programme	
Part	Progression point	Part	Progression point
Part 1	End of year 1	Part 1	End of 8 months
Part 2	End of year 2	Part 2	End of 16 months
Part 3	End of year 3	Part 3	End of 24 months

All universities will have developed guidance to supporting students on practice placement. Building on the work of the Pan London PAD for pre-registration nursing students to meet Future Nurse: Standards of Proficiency for Registered Nurses (NMC 2018a), Health Education England supported the development of an England PAD for nursing associates. The nursing associate document was developed using a similar framework to the Pan London PAD; however, the content reflects the requirements of the NMC's standards of proficiency for nursing associates (NMC 2018c). Within the nursing associate programmes, there are additional requirements for apprenticeships that are specific to individual universities and are not uniform.

Go online

- Sample versions of the Pan London pre-registration practice assessment document for student nurses can be accessed via the Pan London Practice Learning Group website: https://plplg.uk/plpad-2-0
- Sample versions of the England practice assessment document for nursing associates can be accessed via the Pan London Practice Learning Group website: https://plplg.uk/nursing-associates

The Pan London Practice Learning Group has developed a guide to using the PAD, which can be found on the group's website. This is a comprehensive step by step guide and includes background information in relation to Future Nurse: Standards of Proficiency (NMC 2018a), a summary of all the component parts of the PAD outlined in this chapter, criteria for assessment, the responsibilities of the students and others in relation to the PAD regarding supporting and assessing students in practice. There is also a guide to using the PAD for nursing associate programmes on the website.

Go online

- The guide to using the PAD for pre-registration nursing programmes can be accessed via the Pan London Practice Learning Group website: https://plplg.uk/wp-content/uploads/2019/06/Guide-to-using-PLPAD-2.0-JF-NF-Validation-Final-11.2.19.pdf

- The guide to using the england nursing associate PAD for nursing associate programmes can be accessed via the Pan London Practice Learning Group website: https://plplg.uk/wp-content/uploads/2019/06/Guide-to-using-the-England-NA-PAD-JF-NF-Final-7.5.19.pdf

Complete this activity now

Look at your Practice Assessment Document. Familiarise yourself with the components in your PAD as listed below.

Components of practice assessment document	
Guidance for using the PAD	Medicines management
Criteria for assessment in practice	Patient/service user/carer feedback
Initial interview	Record of working with and learning from others/interprofessional working
Orientation	Record of communication/additional feedback
Professional values in practice	Record of peer feedback
Mid-point interview and final interview	Record of practice hours
Assessment of proficiencies	Ongoing achievement record
Episode(s) of care	Action plan

How do these components relate to some of the theory and skills-based sessions you have been covering in your university-based classes?

Assessment in practice

Assessment is not only about whether the student has achieved a specific proficiency or skill, but is also a process that should incorporate both formative and summative assessment that strongly influences the overall learning and includes the related support to enable a student's development towards registration (Boud and Molloy 2013).

Formative assessment

The Quality Assurance Agency for Higher Education defines formative assessment as a developmental process (Quality Assurance Agency for Higher Education 2018) that informs students about outcomes and provides them with feedback to understand strengths, progress, and areas for improvement. Formative assessment will guide you towards how to learn what you need to learn. The continuing feedback on your performance from your practice supervisor and your mid-way interview is an example of formative assessment. You will also have a formative episode of care within your part 1 PAD to encourage you to gain knowledge and skills and seek feedback from your practice supervisor.

Summative assessment

Summative assessment is used to indicate the extent of a student's success in meeting the assessment criteria to gauge the intended learning outcomes of a module or course. This usually occurs at the end of the placement when your practice assessor makes a final decision about your overall achievements against the criteria in the PAD. Typically within a summative assessment, the marks awarded count towards the final mark of the course/module/award; for example, some universities grade their practice assessment while others award a pass.

Those involved in assessment

The key roles for supporting supervision and assessment in practice are the:

- practice supervisor
- practice assessor
- academic assessor.

Practice supervisors, practice assessors and academic assessors have an important role in supporting and guiding you through your learning experience. This includes facilitating any reasonable adjustments you may require to achieve the maximum benefit from the placement. As well as undertaking the required assessments, the roles of the practice supervisor and practice assessor also include identifying relevant learning opportunities and creating learning and development plans with you. A brief outline of these roles is included here:

- Practice supervisors are registered nurses or midwives or registered health and social care professionals.
- Practice assessors are registered nurses with current knowledge and expertise and are appropriately prepared for the role.
- Academic assessors are registered nurses and are nominated for each part of the programme and are appropriately prepared for the role. This is usually a member of the universities link lecturer team who has a wider role in supporting the team in a specific practice area in their learning and assessment role.

Criteria for assessment in practice

Within the PAD, three key statements have been developed to reflect the level of performance that you are required to demonstrate by the end of each part, as well as the level of assistance that may be required during the part. By the end of the part, you should be practising independently, competently and confidently. The three levels of performance to be met by the end of each part are shown in Table 9.2.

TABLE 9.2

The three levels of performance to be met by the end of each part.

By the end of Part 1	Guided participation in care and performing with increasing confidence and competence
By the end of Part 2	Active participation in care with minimal guidance and performing with increased confidence and competence
By the end of Part 3	Practicing independently with minimal supervision and leading and coordinating care with confidence

At the end of each part, your level of performance will be assessed against a specified set of criteria related to knowledge, skills, attitudes and values. These criteria are used to assess you on different placements across the year as you work towards the overall performance level to be achieved by the end of the part (Table 9.2).

If your performance gives cause for concern at the mid-point interview, feedback must be given and an action plan developed to enable you to work on the areas identified prior to the final interview (discussed later in this chapter). The practice assessor must communicate with and involve your nominated academic assessor in this process.

Price et al. (2012) discuss the importance of students and staff being assessment literate and define this concept of 'assessment literacy' as involving an appreciation of the purposes and processes of assessment. Within the PAD there are guidelines relating to how the assessment is managed within each university, and you should ensure that you have read and understood them. You should take responsibility for your own learning and know how to access support.

Hear it from the student

I am a second year adult nursing student and the best advice I was given was to spend time going through my PAD prior to going on placement for the first time and prior to each placement. This enables me to familiarise myself with what is expected of me on placement, what I need to be assessed on, to begin to think about what goals I want to set for myself on my next placement and to think about the learning opportunities that may be available for me to discuss at my initial interview with my practice assessor/practice supervisor.

It is also useful to review the ongoing achievement record, which is a summary of all my placements over the duration of the programme (two or three years, depending on the programme). Reflecting on my achievements to date in my programme can help me identify what is still required to achieve as part of my practice assessment requirements on placement. Preparation and planning what I want to get out of my practice placement can enable me to achieve more out of my practice. Next year, I will be using an electronic PAD and so will need to fully understand how this works for both myself and my practice supervisor and practice assessors.

Complete this activity before your next placement

Look at the components of your PAD. Some examples are given below of what you may wish to discuss in relation to some components.

PAD component	What do I need to do?
Initial interview	• What do I want to discuss with my practice assessor/practice supervisor in my initial interview? • What goals do I want to achieve as part of my learning? • What learning opportunities are there for me on this placement? • What do I need to be assessed on? (e.g. year 2 student: on this placement I need to practice medicines management and undertake/pass episode of care 1)
Mid-point interview	• I need to get more opportunities to practice medicines. • I will be more proactive in seeking learning opportunities with other members of the multidisciplinary team.
Year 2: episode of care 1	To discuss with my practice assessor the opportunity to undertake a formative episode of care by mid placement and the summative episode of care by the end of placement.
Learning and development plan	To discuss how to set SMART objectives as I find it challenging to be realistic and not set too many goals that I find difficult to achieve.
Getting feedback	To be more proactive in seeking feedback from other members of the multidisciplinary team that I work with and to request they feedback on the forms available in the PAD.

Components of the practice assessment document

Initial interview

The initial interview can be completed by a practice supervisor or practice assessor. If it is completed by the practice supervisor, they must discuss and agree with the practice assessor. This meeting should take place within the first week of the placement. It is not an interview in the sense of you being asked a number of direct questions; it should be centred around a discussion regarding your learning and development needs to enable you to get the best out of your placement.

Go online

An initial interview podcast developed by the Pan London Practice Learning Group is available from, https://plplg.uk/sssa-resources

What are the key points you have learned from the podcast in relation to preparing for orientation?

As a year 1 student on a first placement, you could consider what theory and practice you have undertaken within the university setting. For example, this might relate to communication skills, the NMC Code (NMC 2018d) or specific clinical skills that you have practised within the university and hence need to extend your understanding and gain further practice. It is important that you link these skills to some of the proficiencies or professional values in your Part 1 PAD. You need to consider the available learning opportunities within your allocated area and take these into consideration.

The welcome pack or orientation pack for your practice area will help you to plan. It is expected that students will have undertaken some preparation in advance of starting a placement, although for a first or second placement when you are not so familiar with healthcare, your practice supervisor/practice assessor will guide you. It is expected in all situations that you then work with your practice supervisor/practice assessor to negotiate and agree an appropriate learning plan.

Placement orientation

A structured orientation is key to providing students with a meaningful and valuable learning experience (Quinlivan et al. 2019) and a general introduction to the health and social care placement setting is an important requirement for the student's safety and the safety of others.

Within the PAD, the orientation checklist requires you to have an overview and explanation of health and safety policies, fire procedures, resuscitation policy procedures and equipment shown, so that you know what to do in an emergency and your role, which will depend on your level of experience.

Other information will include shift times, mealtimes and reporting sick policies, policy regarding safeguarding process and raising concerns, all which may also be included in your welcome pack and form part of understanding your professional role in practice.

You will note that risk assessments and reasonable adjustments must be discussed and again this is to ensure the staff in practice understand your requirements that may relate to disability, learning or pregnancy needs, but practice staff can only act and support if you have shared this information with them, which we encourage you to do (see also Chapter 4).

Completing your orientation

Within the PAD, the orientation form may be completed and signed by the practice supervisor, practice assessor or any registered health care professional, although another member of the team may also support aspects of the process. For example, an experienced healthcare assistant may show you around the area and/or a senior student peer could direct you to the welcome pack and introduce you to local policies, but a registered staff member, nurse or nursing associate would be the most appropriate person to discuss the application of these policies, discuss any reasonable adjustments you may require, raising concerns and your own professional role within the team. Most of the orientation checklist should be completed on your first day, although there may be a small number of items not completed until day 2. Note that there are also a couple of items which are only required when needed – for example, prior to the use of certain devices/equipment within the area.

The Strengthening Team-based Education in Practice (Figure 9.1) is an example of a best practice guide for orientation, and is a useful summary of what an orientation should include (STEP Project Team 2020).

WHAT SHOULD AN ORIENTATION INCLUDE? A best practice guide

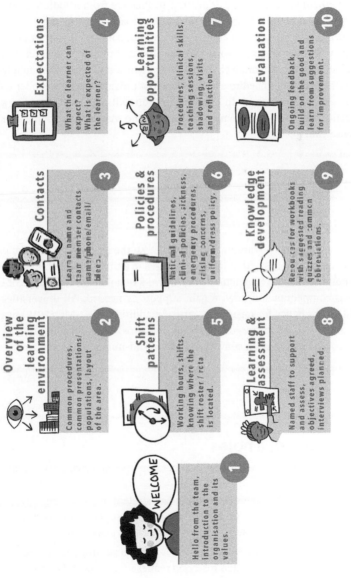

1 WELCOME
Hello from the team, introduction to the organisation and its values.

2 Overview of the learning environment
Common procedures, common presentations/ populations, layout of the area.

3 Contacts
Learner name and team member contacts name/phone/email/ bleep.

4 Expectations
What the learner can expect? What is expected of the learner?

5 Shift patterns
Working hours, shifts, knowing where the shift roster / rota is located.

6 Policies & procedures
National guidelines, clinical policies, sickness, emergency procedures, raising concerns, uniform/dress policy.

7 Learning opportunities
Procedures, clinical skills, teaching sessions, shadowing, visits and reflection.

8 Learning & assessment
Named staff to support and assess, objectives agreed, interviews planned.

9 Knowledge development
Resources for workbooks with suggested reading quizzes and common abbreviations.

10 Evaluation
Ongoing feedback, build on the good and learn from suggestions for improvement.

twitter - @STEPMDX

**FIGURE 9.1 Summary of orientation – best practice. *Source:* STEP (2020) Strengthening Team-based Education in Practice. Middlesex University (https://www.stepapproach-learning.org).

Go online

Strengthening Team-based Education in Practice from Middlesex University is a best practice guide: www.stepapproach-learning.org

If by day 2 of your placement you have not completed your orientation, you must speak to your practice assessor/practice supervisor, if available, or the person in charge, and agree how and when to complete it. Otherwise, you need to escalate this to a university staff member or your academic assessor. In many areas, you will also have access to a practice educator or placement facilitator who may be able to guide or advise you.

Green flag

Ensure that you are familiar with and know the policy for raising and escalating concerns within the practice area in a timely manner. It is also important that you understand your university policy for reporting concerns/complaints and how to gain support as needed. All universities will have a policy for raising concerns. In addition, the NMC (2019) has guidance on the process for raising concerns: www.nmc.org.uk/standards/guidance/raising-concerns-guidance-for-nurses-and-midwives

A supervisor's notes

(These notes below are applicable to both practice supervisors and practice assessors.)

You have been allocated a second-year student for their eight-week placement. Here is a list of my tips as a practice supervisor to pass on to other staff who supervise and assess students on placement:

- Communicate with your student prior to them starting placement; introduce yourself, discuss rostering requests/requirements, and allocate off duty. Explain how you will work with the student – for example how many shifts in a week.
- Send the student welcome pack to the student in advance of the placement.

- At initial interview, discuss the student's expectations and the expectations of the nursing team while the student is on the placement. You may find it helpful to refer to the professional values in the PAD for this discussion.

- Ensure that your student is aware of the 'nominated person' and the process to escalate concerns.

- Discuss the learning opportunities available on placement and encourage the student to take responsibility for their learning, with supervision. Help the student to identify SMART objectives in their initial learning and development plan.

- Encourage the student to seek oral and written feedback from other nurses and members of the multidisciplinary team they have worked with.

- Identify with the student what they need to achieve on placement in relation to their programme and PAD (i.e. specific proficiencies they need to complete, medicines management assessments or complete an episode of care).

- Are there any areas previously identified on other placements which the student needs to develop further (e.g. communication skills)?

- Are there any areas within professional values on which the student could benefit from focusing?

- Discuss with student who to contact in the event of issues which may arise on placement.

Mid-point interview

The mid-point interview is an essential and critical component of assessment. This is your opportunity to reflect on your experience and achievements and seek feedback on your performance from the practice assessor.

The first section that needs completing on the midway feedback form is student's self-assessment/reflection on progress. This provides you with the opportunity to consider your overall progression referring to your personal learning needs, professional values and proficiencies.

As a student, you need to identify your strengths and document areas for development. Consider what experiences you have had to date and how these relate to the proficiencies/skills in your PAD and your overall development and confidence.

It is important to refer back to the criteria set out for each part and review your knowledge, skills, attitudes and values; for example, in Part 2 the level of performance expected is that a student should demonstrate:

Active participation in care with minimal guidance and increasing confidence

As you can see from Table 9.3, you are expected to be able to provide a rationale to support care delivery, so it is important to continually be questioning why you are doing things and how they benefit the individual in your care.

Practice assessor's comments

The practice assessor is required to discuss with the student their self-assessment and comment on their progression, again using the criteria for assessment/practice descriptors in Table 9.3 detailing

---

TABLE 9.3

Levels of participation.

Achieved	Knowledge	Skills	Attitude and values
YES	Has a sound knowledge base to support safe and effective practice and provide the rationale to support decision making.	Utilises a range of skills to deliver safe, person centred and evidence-based care with increased confidence and in a range of contexts.	Demonstrates an understanding of professional roles and responsibilities within the multidisciplinary team. Maximises opportunities to extend own knowledge.
NO	Has a superficial knowledge base and is unable to provide a rationale for care, demonstrating unsafe practice?	With supervision is not able to demonstrate safe practice and is unable to perform the activity and/or follow instructions despite repeated guidance.	Demonstrates lack of self-awareness and understanding of professional role and responsibilities. Is not asking appropriate questions nor engaged with their own learning.

evidence used to inform their decision. The evidence may be related to what the practice assessor observed when working with a specific student or may be based on feedback from practice supervisors. If the practice assessor has any concerns, they are expected to raise them with the academic assessor and consider whether an action plan would support the student's development and progression. Action plans are discussed later in the chapter.

Learning and development needs

Within your PAD, you are required to identify your learning and development needs on placement in the initial interview and mid-point interview. Writing objectives to facilitate your learning using SMART principles will enable you to identify your learning needs and have specific goals to work towards and achieve during your placement. SMART is an acronym for specific, measurable, achievable, realistic and timebound (Table 9.4).

TABLE **9.4**

SMART goals.

SMART goals	What does this mean?
Specific	Specific goals are more effective as they help you outline the steps you need to achieve them. Use specific terms and be clear with what you want to achieve and enable you to focus.
Measurable	What evidence will you need to know that you have completed your goal? Quantifying your goals makes them more tangible and can be measured.
Achievable	Setting a reasonable target is key. If it is too ambitious this can be overwhelming and if too easy will limit you achieving your full potential.
Realistic	Within reach and relevant
Timebound	Set a realistic timeframe to complete your goal. A deadline will help you focus.

Hear it from the student

In this video clip, Ben Low, 'the London Nurse' gives tips and guidance for first-year students on how to make your objectives SMART: https://www.youtube.com/watch?v=tso3qt7z3ZM

Examples of SMART objectives identified within the video clip include:

'By week 6 of my placement I would like to become competent at taking and documenting temperature, manual pulse, respiratory rate and blood pressure on the defined age range of patients, ensuring that I report findings to the nurse that I am working with.'

'To carry out a full admission completing paperwork and orientating the patient and family to the clinical environment with staff I am working with by midpoint, and then complete a full admission by the end of placement.'

'During my eight-week placement I would like to work on my confidence and skills at communicating with patients and their families within the clinical environment, being able to gain a greater understanding of professional boundaries and clinical practice on a daily basis with the patients I am caring for.'

Try this on placement

On your next placement, in your *initial interview*, identify your learning and development needs using SMART goals and discuss and agree these with your practice assessor.

At your *mid-point interview*, review your learning and development needs and SMART goals set at Initial Interview.

- Are you 'on track' to meet your goals on this placement?
- Do you need to amend any of your goals?
- Do you need to seek out further learning opportunities on placement to help you meet your learning needs and achieve your goals?

At your *final interview*, review your SMART goals.

- Did you achieve all your goals?
- What have you learned from goal setting and reviewing your goals with your practice assessor?
- Would you do anything differently on your next placement in relation to goal setting?

Professional values

As a student, you are expected to demonstrate high standards of professional conduct at all times during your practice placements. You should work within the ethical and legal frameworks and be able to articulate the underpinning values of the NMC Code (NMC 2018d).

The professional values reflect several proficiency statements and are captured under the four sections of the Code (NMC 2018d). All four must be achieved by the end of each placement. As the student, you are required to select one example from your practice on each placement to demonstrate how you practice within the Code. Confidentiality in relation to people receiving care and service providers must be maintained.

Who assesses the professional values?

The practice supervisor or practice assessor can assess your mid-point professional values. If the practice supervisor assesses the mid-point, this must be reviewed and agreed by your practice assessor. The final professional values on each placement are assessed by the practice assessor, who will discuss and review your reflection with you. If there are any concerns raised regarding your level of performance these should be discussed with your academic assessor.

Where other components have been assessed and achieved (e.g. a proficiency assessed at the beginning of the part), you need to demonstrate continued competence and confidence in the proficiency. Professional value statement 8: 'The student makes a consistent effort to engage in the requisite standards of care and learning based on best available evidence' enables the assessor to ensure and record that the student is meeting this requirement. When setting learning outcomes for your placement and you consider that you need further rehearsal in some proficiencies, you can discuss this with your practice assessor and agree ways in which this may be achieved on placement.

As the student, you are required to select one example from your practice on each placement to demonstrate how you practice within the Code. Again, confidentiality in relation to people receiving care and service providers should be maintained. For each placement, a different area of the Code should be selected to reflect on. The professional values show progressions through Parts 1–3.

Try this on placement

In the NMC Code (NMC 2018d), there are four sections:

1. Prioritise people
2. Practise effectively
3. Preserve safety
4. Promote professionalism and trust.

Select one example from your recent practice placement to demonstrate how you practice within the NMC Code and write a short reflection.

How has this influenced your practice?

Proficiencies

As presented in Chapter 2, the NMC Future Nurse: Standards of Proficiency for Registered Nurses are outlined. These proficiencies 'specify the knowledge and skills that registered nurses must demonstrate when caring for people of all ages and across all care settings' (NMC 2018b, p. 3). These proficiencies are incorporated into seven platforms; for example, platform 1 is 'being an accountable professional' and platform 7 is 'coordinating care'. In addition to the proficiencies, there are a number of skills and nursing procedures that also must be met during the programme. These include the 'communication and relationship management skills', which form Annexe A and the 'nursing procedures', which form Annexe B of the standards.

Within the PAD, the skills and nursing procedures have been blended with the proficiencies and there are approximately 30 of these combined proficiencies to be met in each part of the PAD.

These proficiencies 'apply to all registered nurses but the level of expertise and knowledge required will vary depending on the chosen field(s) of practice' (NMC 2018b, pp. 22, 26). Guidance on the meaning and interpretation of this statement will be provided by your programme team within your university.

Assessment of proficiencies is undertaken across the part. These proficiencies can be assessed in a range of placements but need to be assessed as achieved (YES) at least once by the end of the part. If a proficiency is assessed as achieved (YES) early in the part, it is expected that you maintain that level of competence and can be reassessed in subsequent placements at the practice assessor's discretion. Some of the proficiencies may be met within simulated learning, in line with NMC requirements and the individual university's policy.

To support your progress effectively through the programme and in using the valuable opportunities available across a range of placements, certain proficiencies have been identified that can be met in Part 2 *or* Part 3 of the programme. These are listed in the Part 2 and Part 3 documents and the ongoing achievement record (OAR). The practice assessor needs to complete this at the end of Part 2 and Part 3. Any proficiencies not met in Part 2 are then identified as your needing to achieve them in Part 3.

Complete this activity now

Review the following proficiencies (as appropriate) and consider how they could be achieved in practice. Consider the theoretical knowledge that may be required to underpin understanding the proficiency and how you would demonstrate achievement in practice:

Part 1 proficiency 3: Accurately processes all information gathered during the assessment process to identify needs for fundamental nursing care and develop and document person-centred care plans.

Part 2 proficiency 22: Provide information and explanation to people, families and carers and responds appropriately to questions about their treatment and care.

Part 3: proficiency 19: Effectively manages and prioritises the care needs of a group of people demonstrating appropriate communication and leadership skills to delegate responsibility for care to others in the team as required.

The following sections provide examples of how these proficiencies could be achieved in practice.

Part 1 proficiency 3

Accurately processes all information gathered during the assessment process to identify needs for fundamental nursing care and develop and document person-centred care plans.

This proficiency could be demonstrated via any patient/service user interaction and within any field of practice. It may be that you have been allocated to work with a specific individual you have not previously met, and you will undertake your own assessment. You may need to consider the level of support the individual needs. Do they need help with mobilising, with communication, with personal hygiene? How can you work with this individual/family/carer to promote self-care/independence? as appropriate.

Part 2 proficiency 22

Provide information and explanation to people, families and carers and responds appropriately to questions about their treatment and care.

In this situation, you need to ensure that you are working within your scope of practice and you are providing accurate and timely information. It may be about diet, treatment or medication. This should have previously been discussed with a member of staff or your practice supervisor/practice assessor to ensure that you are providing correct guidance. They can provide the level of supervision deemed necessary. You may need to refer to a member of staff within the area to address any queries regarding treatment and care.

Part 3 proficiency 19

Effectively manages and prioritises the care needs of a group of people demonstrating appropriate communication and leadership skills to delegate responsibility for care to others in the team as required.

You will have been building your communication and leadership skills across the programme and through managing the care for a small group of patients/service users you will be expected to appropriately prioritise their care needs, work as a member of the team.

Within the PAD, there are some proficiencies/skills that may be more challenging to meet in certain fields of practice. For example, for pre-registration students in mental health and learning disability fields, proficiencies in relation to physical skills including the management of nasogastric tubes, electrocardiograms, intravenous therapy and chest auscultation may be difficult to achieve. As per the NMC guidance it is important to emphasise that, where possible, student assessment should occur within the practice setting. However, it is acknowledged that this may not always be achievable in all fields of nursing owing to the nature of the service and the model of care delivery. Universities across the country may have developed guidance to support the achievement of Future Nurse: Standards of Proficiency (NMC 2018a).

Go online

Visit the Pan London Practice Learning Group website for some guidance regarding completion of specific proficiencies – a process agreed across London: https://plplg.uk/further resources/#Assessment

Episodes of care

This holistic assessment(s) facilitates and demonstrates your progress and must be achieved by the end of each part. The episodes of care reflect Future Nurse standards of proficiency and complexity and changing health care environments where care delivery takes place (NMC 2018a) – that is, integrated health and social care settings.

Students in discussion with their practice assessor should identify the appropriate placement and episode of care to complete this assessment. As there is only one opportunity for assessment, the planning should take this into consideration to maximise the learning for the student.

- Part 1 – there is one episode of care that you need to be assessed on by your practice assessor. This is a summative assessment. However, you are encouraged to complete one as a formative assessment and this can be undertaken with your practice supervisor. This episode of care involves meeting the needs of an individual person receiving care.
- Part 2 – there are two episodes of care in Part 2 to facilitate the development of knowledge and skills related to your field of practice.
  - Episode 1 – this involves the care of a group of people receiving care or an individual with complex care needs.

- ○ Episode 2 – this involves the care of a group of people receiving care with increasingly complex health and social care needs.
- Part 3 – there are two episodes of care in Part 3 to facilitate the development and consolidation of knowledge and skills related to your field of practice.
  - ○ Episode of care 1 – supervising and teaching a junior learner in practice, based on the delivery of direct person-centred care.
  - ○ Episode of care 2 – organisation and management of care for a group/caseload of people with complex care covering all seven platforms.

Within each episode of care, there is specific guidance to help you reflect on your practice in relation to the delivery of person-centred care and could include what you did well, what you would do differently and what learning from each episode of care could be transferred to other areas of practice.

Medicines management

Assessments of medicines management can be carried out in any setting where there is regular dispensing and administration of medicines to individuals or groups, either in the student's field of practice or in any other experiential placement. The level of complexity is enhanced each year/part. The practice assessor will agree with you when this should be undertaken.

There is one assessment included in each part and each must be achieved by the end of the part. You and your practice assessor should identify the appropriate placement to complete this assessment. By the end of Part 3, you should be consolidating your knowledge, skills and competence in relation to the safe administration of medicines within the required regulatory frameworks relating to Future Nurse (NMC 2018a), the Code (NMC 2018d) and *A Competency Framework for all Prescribers* (Royal Pharmaceutical Society 2021).

In discussion with your practice assessor, as a student you should identify the appropriate placement to complete this assessment. As there is only one opportunity for assessment the planning should take this into consideration to maximise your learning. You should be allowed a number of practice opportunities to administer medicines under supervision prior to undertaking the medicines management assessment. Dispensing, administering and management of medicines is an integral part of nursing care. Practice staff should facilitate regular opportunities for their students to practice medicines management on all placements where appropriate.

Patient/service user/carer feedback form

Feedback should be sought in relation to how you have cared for the person receiving care. This is not formally assessed but will make an important contribution to your overall feedback. The evaluation of the first Pan London PAD highlighted what patients valued in their care and positive feedback helped to build students' confidence, self-esteem, is motivating and rewarding (Baillie and Fish 2021).

Within each placement there is a page for you to receive feedback directly from someone you have cared for and/or carers. In some PADs, a range of formats are provided. The practice supervisor/practice assessor should obtain consent from patients/service users/carers to complete the form and they should feel able to decline to participate and sign the form on completion. It may not be possible to have this completed in every placement.

Feedback as part of the assessment process

Receiving feedback on your professional values and behaviour, the care you deliver and how you interact and communicate with members of the team, the patients in your care and their relatives/carers is integral to the assessment process on your practice placements. Establishing a feedback routine and being proactive can enable you to get a range of feedback from those you work with and who supervise you.

Providing your own feedback on what you have achieved and where you need to learn/gain confidence is an important part of your learning. This is most commonly undertaken through reflecting on your practice overall or on the shift you have just worked and on specific aspects of learning that you may be focusing on. For example, this could be reflecting on caring for a group of three patients with minimal prompting; how you have communicated an aspect of care with the patient and their carer in relation to how they manage their diabetes or how you have interacted with a patient who is refusing treatment due to their anxiety and prior experience.

Over to you
How to get feedback on placement

- Be proactive in seeking feedback.
- Timing of when you ask for feedback matters – be aware of what is going on in the practice area and try to ask for feedback at what appears to be an appropriate time for both you and your practice supervisor/practice assessor (this will not necessarily be at the end of a busy shift).
- Take ownership of your learning experience.
- Reflect on your own learning, ensuring confidentiality is maintained, and share your reflections with your practice assessor/supervisor.
- Seek feedback from others you have worked with in the multidisciplinary team, other nurses, health care assistants, peers, and patients/carers. Use the appropriate documentation in the PAD to get others to record their feedback.

Additional feedback on practice placement

Within the PAD, there are opportunities for others to contribute feedback on your practice in addition to your practice supervisor and practice assessor. This may include other nurses you have worked with, health care assistants, members of the multidisciplinary team including allied health professionals, patients/service users/carers and peers.

Recording of working with and learning from others/ interprofessional working

You will have opportunities across all parts to work with other professions across a range of teams and agencies and will be able to gain an understanding of the different roles and responsibilities and importance of teamwork in providing person centred care.

You should reflect on your learning when working with members of the multidisciplinary team and document this. The practice supervisor will discuss your reflection and give feedback. The practice assessor will review documented records where you have worked with other health and social care professionals and incorporate their feedback into assessment where appropriate.

There will also be opportunities where carers are involved in care delivery that you can learn from. For example, parents caring for their child with long term conditions such as cystic fibrosis, carers supporting a relative with dementia in a variety of care settings including the person's own home or a nursing home or managing a patient with a mental health condition such as anxiety. As students working alongside carers, you can gain insight and learning from them and their experiences.

Over to you

Identify a patient you have cared for where the patient's carer(s) has been integral to their management and care (remember you must adhere to the rules of confidentiality)

- What did you learn from the patient's carer(s)?

- What do nurses need to consider when supporting carers?

Record of communication and additional feedback

These records can be completed by practice supervisors, practice assessors, academic assessors, or any other members of the team involved in your supervision and assessment. This is for additional feedback that has not previously been documented in the PAD (i.e. other students who have worked alongside you or have had the opportunity to discuss your learning needs with you). If you have facilitated a teaching session on placement you can use this form to obtain feedback.

Record of peer feedback

Peer feedback forms have been introduced into the PAD to enhance the potential for student support and learning with peer support being identified as having mutual benefits for both the giver and the receiver (Morley 2015; Wilson et al. 2019).

In Parts 2 and 3 you are encouraged to obtain feedback from your student peers (i.e. other students who have worked alongside you or have had the opportunity to discuss your learning needs with you). For example, if you have facilitated a teaching session on placement you can use this form to obtain feedback. Feedback is an essential part of the learning process. Through engaging in peer review and receiving feedback from a number of peers it is an opportunity for you to be exposed to a wider diversity of perspectives as well as giving students the opportunity to develop their skills in peer review and feedback (NMC 2018a).

Complete this activity now
Peer learning

You are a Part 3 student nurse and will be working together with a Part 2 student nurse for the next two shifts. You would like to use this as an opportunity to facilitate learning with the student.

How will you prepare for this to facilitate peer support and learning?

What knowledge and skills can you gain from undertaking your peer learning and support role with this Part 2 student?

Ongoing achievement record

The OAR is a separate document that summarises your achievements in each placement and with the PAD provides a comprehensive record of your professional development and performance in practice. You are responsible for the safekeeping and maintenance of your PAD and OAR. It should be available to your practice supervisor, practice assessor and academic assessor at all times when you are in placement together with the OAR.

The practice assessor completes the summary page at the end of each placement and at the end of each part completes the progression statement. The academic assessor confirms the completion of each placement, adds comments and at the end of each part completes the progression statement. Any proficiencies not met in Part 2 are then identified and recorded to enable you as being required to achieve these proficiencies in Part 3.

Action plan

Chapter 10 focuses on receiving feedback, feed forward and action plans. Action plans are discussed briefly here as they are an integral part of the PAD. Obtaining feedback is a priority on practice placements.

> ### Go online
>
> Never fail! How to confidently overcome action plans, a video from the London Nurse, gives lots of tips on how to get feedback and establish a feedback routine: https://www.youtube.com/watch?v=WtFrU1LX8A4

If your performance and/or progress causes concern, then an action plan enables you to focus on the areas which you need to work on. Your practice assessor will liaise with academic assessors who will work together to support you. The practice assessor will monitor performance. SMART objectives should be used to develop the action plan (Figure 9.2). Refer to earlier guidance within this chapter on how to write objectives using SMART principles. Providing opportunities for you as a student to engage in learning while providing support will enable you to achieve the action plan.

Electronic practice assessment document

Many universities now use an online platform to document their practice assessment rather than paper documentation. There are a range of platforms for delivering the e-PAD, including PARE, pebble PAD, Axia Digital, and ARC.

In London, many universities are using MyKnowledgeMap and are at various stages of introducing and implementing this online platform. The e-PAD, being digital and multiplatform, increases usability. It promotes ease of access through innovative and intuitive technology and the e-PAD has improved transparency, accountability and processes in supporting students through their journey to qualification (PLPLG 2021).

Action Plan

An action plan is required when a student's performance causes concern

The practice assessor must liaise with the academic assessor and the senior practice representative

The **SMART** principles should be used to construct the action plan.

Placement name:			Date action plan initiated:	
Nature of concern Refer to professional value(s), proficiency and/or episode of care (specific)	**What does the student need to demonstrate?** Objectives and measure of success (measurable, achievable and realistic)	**Support available and who is responsible**	**Date for review** (timed)	**Review/feedback**
				Date:
				Comments:
Student's name:		Signature:	Date:	Practice assessor's name:
Practice assessor's name:		Signature:	Date:	
Academic assessor's name:		Signature:	Date:	Signature:

FIGURE 9.2 Action plan.

Go online

Look up the resources to support the introduction and implementation of the Pan London e-PAD for students and staff: https://plplg.uk/pan-london-epad

Record of practice hours

Students are required to provide evidence of having completed the required number of practice hours for NMC registration. A range of staff members need to verify the practice hours on the form. These include the practice assessor, practice supervisor, ward manager, and/or a member of the education team on placement who must verify the student's hours at the end of each shift/week on the appropriate form. Specific information is provided from your university regarding how your practice hours are reported and recorded.

Your role in supporting your learning in practice

As a student, you have a key role in supporting your supervision and assessment in practice and in enhancing the learning environment and can do this by:

- Demonstrating high standards of professional conduct at all times and be able to articulate the underpinning values of the Code (NMC 2018d).
- Being prepared for and have a sound understanding of the proficiencies/skills you need to achieve, and processes related to using your e-PAD where appropriate.
- Contacting the area in advance to ensure you are familiar with the location and your allocated shifts/duties.
- Being aware of the name of the person you should speak to in the practice area if you have concerns.
- Actively seeking out practice supervisors to support your learning and encourage feedback to be recorded in your PAD.
- Knowing the name of your nominated practice assessor and your academic assessor from the beginning of the placement.
- Understanding the support services available both within the practice area and via the university while in practice.
- Reflecting regularly on your learning in practice and support the learning of others.
- Raising concerns promptly and seeking support as required.
- Providing feedback on your learning experience both in the placement area and on return to the university to support monitoring and enhancement of the learning environment.

- If you have a paper PAD, always keep your PAD and OAR with you when you are on practice placement.
- Enjoy your practice placement and remember there is always someone available to provide support and guidance.

Acknowledgements

The second Pan London PAD was developed by the Pan London Practice Learning Group, Kathy Wilson (Chair), Nicki Fowler (Vice Chair) in collaboration with practice partners, mentors, academic staff, students and service users across the London region, with wider consultation across all regions in England.

References

Baillie, L. and Fish, J. (2021). An evaluation of a unified practice assessment document for student nurses: students', mentors' and academics' views and experiences. *Journal of Practice Teaching and Learning* 18 (1–2): 24–37.

Boud, D. and Molloy, E. (2013). Rethinking models of feedback for learning: the challenge of design. *Assessment and Evaluation in Higher Education* 38 (6): 698–712.

Lauder, W., Roxburgh, M., Holland, K., et al (2008). *Nursing and Midwifery in Scotland: Being Fit for Practice*. The Report of the Evaluation of Fitness for Practice Pre-Registration Nursing and Midwifery Curricula Project. Edinburgh: NHS Education Scotland.

Morley, D. (2015). *A Grounded Theory Study Exploring First Year Student Nurses' Learning in Practice*. PhD thesis. Bournemouth: Bournemouth University.

NHS Education for Scotland (2011). *Developing a National Approach to Practice Assessment Documentation for the Pre-Registration Nursing Programmes in.* Edinburgh: NHS Education for Scotland.

Nursing and Midwifery Council (2018a). *Future Nurse: Standards of Proficiency for Registered Nurses.* London: NMC www.nmc.org.uk/globalassets/sitedocuments/standards-of-proficiency/nurses/future-nurse-proficiencies.pdf (accessed July 2022).

Nursing and Midwifery Council (2018b). *Realising Professionalism: Standards for Education and Training Part 2: Standards for Student Supervision and Assessment.* London: NMC www.nmc.org.uk/globalassets/sitedocuments/standards-of-proficiency/standards-for-student-supervision-and-assessment/student-supervision-assessment.pdf (accessed July 2022).

Nursing and Midwifery Council (2018c). *Standards of Proficiency for Nursing Associates.* London: NMC www.nmc.org.uk/standards/standards-for-nursing-associates/standards-of-proficiency-for-nursing-associates (accessed July 2022).

Nursing and Midwifery Council (2018d). *The Code: Professional Standards of Practice and Behaviour for Nurses, Midwives and Nursing Associates (Updated from 2015)*. London: NMC www.nmc.org.uk/globalassets/sitedocuments/nmc-publications/nmc-code.pdf (accessed July 2022).

Nursing and Midwifery Council (2019). *Raising Concerns Guidance for Nurses, Midwives and Nursing Associates*. London: NMC www.nmc.org.uk/globalassets/blocks/media-block/raising-concerns-v2.pdf (accessed July 2022).

Pan London Practice Learning Group (2021). *Pan London e-PAD: project update*. PLPLG Newsletter (12). https://plplg.uk/wp-content/uploads/2021/07/PLPLG_Newsletter_A4_Issue-12_v5.pdf

Price, M., Rust, C., O'Donovan, B. et al. (2012). *Assessment Literacy: The Foundation for Improving Student Learning*. Oxford: Oxford Centre for Staff and Learning Development, Oxford Brookes University.

Quality Assurance Agency (2018). *The Revised UK Quality Code for Education*. Gloucester: QAA. www.qaa.ac.uk/the-quality-code# (accessed 18 March 2023).

Quinlivan, L., Sookraj-Bahal, S., Moody, J. et al. (2019). Comprehensive orientation and socialisation. In: *Facilitating Learning in Practice: A research-based approach to challenges and solutions* (ed. D. Morley, K. Wilson, and N. Holbery), 6 17. Oxford: Routledge.

Royal Pharmaceutical Society (2021) *A Competency Framework for all Prescribers*. www.rpharms.com/resources/frameworks/prescribing competency-framework/competency-framework (accessed 18 March 2023).

STEP Project Team (2020). *Strengthening Team-Based Education in Practice*. Middlesex University https://www.stepapproach-learning.org/.

Wilson, K., Cooper, N., and Baron, M. (2019). Student peer support and learning. In: *Facilitating Learning in Practice: A research-based approach to challenges and solutions* (ed. D. Morley, K. Wilson, and N. Holbery), 32 43. Oxford: Routledge.

Receiving feedback and feedforward

Siobhan McGuckin

AIM

This chapter demonstrates the benefits and importance of receiving and giving feedback, both clinically and academically.

LEARNING OUTCOMES

Having read this chapter, you will be able to:

1. Deliver effective, timely feedback.
2. Process the feedback and feedforward in a positive manner.
3. Learn from the feedback and feedforward to enhance both your clinical and academic professional development.
4. Adhere to and work within your scope of practice: the Nursing and Midwifery Council (NMC) Code of Professional Conduct (NMC 2018a).

Succeeding on your Nursing Placement: Supervision, Learning and Assessment for Nursing Students, First Edition. Edited by Ian Peate.
© 2024 John Wiley & Sons Ltd. Published 2024 by John Wiley & Sons Ltd.

Introduction

This chapter explores receiving feedback and the importance of feedforward within clinical environments with placement partners, together with academic feedback from lecturers on individual submitted assignments, open-book examinations, group presentations and multiple-choice question examinations.

How and what we learn from feedback that is given is discussed. What feedback may mean to the student and how receiving feedback can make a person feel are also addressed. The various ways in which feedback can be given are discussed. It is important to remember that not all feedback is negative, but that there are valuable and, at times, constructive lessons to be learnt from the points raised in the feedback. Being partners in the feedback process is essential.

Within any large organisation, and healthcare is no exception, feedback can be delivered in different ways. Feedback will be considered under the following subheadings:

- Compliments and complaints – internal and external to the organisation.
- Action planning to focus upon areas where students are underperforming.

OVER TO YOU

- What is your understanding of feedback and feedforward and its significance?
- Jot down what your experiences have been thus far in your learning journey, in both delivering and receiving feedback and feedforward.
- How did it make you feel?
- Did you feel that your voice was being listened to?

The assessment process and partnerships in feedback

Assessment is an essential aspect of learning, effectively contributing to ensuring that the learning trajectory is continuing and, as such, it is imperative that you are cognisant of what the process involves and its contribution to both feedback and feedforward. This is of utmost importance for all students, but more so for new learners at the beginning of their nursing programmes and the introduction into health and care environments.

Pokorny (2021) informs us that we must be able to differentiate between both assessment of learning and assessment for learning. Simply put, when discussing assessment of learning, there is a focus upon the judging and measuring function of the assessment. Whereas, with assessment for learning, the lecturer can make use of the potential and opportunity to develop, encourage and enhance an in-depth quality driven programme of learning by integrating both assessment and teaching.

So, what does this mean for students and how will it deepen and further develop your knowledge base theoretically and practically? By using this approach, how are you and your team of lecturers going to progress you from where you are now in the learning trajectory to where you need to be by completion of your studies? Sambell et al. (2012) identified six components to assist you not only with your learning but ultimately to be successful (Box 10.1).

When addressing the balance between formative and summative assignments and subsequent feedback, formal studies have emerged from the Transforming the Experience of Students Through Assessment (TESTA) research and change process. The principles underpinning TESTA are that the programme/module teams undertake and view courses holistically by listening to and drawing upon the student's lived experience.

Box 10.1 | Six components that can help students with their learning

- Authentic assessment
- Balancing summative and formative assessment
- Creating opportunities for practice and rehearsal
- Designing formal feedback to improve learning
- Designing opportunities for informal feedback
- Developing students as self-assessors and effective life-long learners

Source: Adapted from Sambell et al. (2012).

> ## Go online
> Access the TESTA website, where you will find a range of resources including case studies: www.testa.ac.uk

However, Jessop (2019) informs us that some students do not see the value in non-contributory formative assessments. Whereas Mc Callum and Milner (2021) suggest that formative assessments can be viewed by some as optional extras. However, King (2022) discusses the positive impact experienced by students of receiving online formative feedback immediately, and how this encouraged and empowered students to take control of their learning and subsequent areas that needed to be developed.

In efforts to enhance and make feedback effective, the Institute for Academic Development (2016), when discussing assessment, invites the person delivering the feedback to be cognisant of the following: to ensure that there is clarity within your feedback, that there is plain and clear signposting as to what the student needs to demonstrate in their next assignment, and also to ensure that feedback is timely (King 2022).

Pokorny and Pickford (2010) state that some students may not, as yet, have identified and mastered the skillset required to carry out self-assessment of their own learning. Gibbs and Simpson (2004) identified research which illustrated that students do not always act upon feedback provided by their lecturers.

Hattie and Timperley (2007) note that feedback is powerful in influencing learning. They also point out that quality feedback contributes to building student's confidence levels. As the student, you need to be supported and given the necessary skill set to enable you to drive feedback for yourself. In efforts to ensure that you are engaged in the process and feel empowered, seek clarification from the lecturer that you have understood the content of the feedback and feedforward processes and for them what/where are the weakest links?

> ## Over to you
> - Do you know how to access your academic feedback?
> - How/where do you receive feedback when on clinical placement?
> - How would you request a meeting with your academic assessor/ practice supervisor or assessor to discuss the feedback?

- Do you always agree/disagree with the feedback provided?
- How does the feedback make you feel? How do you address your feeling in this instance?

Attention needs to be focused on why some students fail to engage with the available feedback that has been presented. Johnson (2013) states that there may be a variety of reasons for not engaging which could include that perhaps students do not find the feedback useful or that the feedback is not sufficiently specific, detailed or individualised.

Hear it from the student

When I was in my first year, I was devastated to learn that I had failed my professional issues assignment, a 2000-word essay. I really worked hard on it, attended the tutorial sessions, and truly gave my heart and soul to it. To receive an F grade shook me to my roots. To make matters worse I was unable to make any sense of the feedback that the marker had given me. I was so despondent, the comments seemed to be unfair.

I picked myself up and made an appointment to see the marker (I was not looking forward to it). When we met, we went through the assignment and the feedback she had given me and, all of a sudden, the penny dropped and I understood where I was going wrong, it was as if someone had turned a light on in a very dark room. I had three weeks left to resubmit, I followed the advice given by the marker and eventually passed the assignment.

I think the feeling of shame, the stress that I could fail again on resubmission, made my anxiety worse, but I did it and with support from my lecturer I passed, albeit a capped grade at 40%, I nevertheless passed.

My advice would be to read the feedback really carefully and seek support as soon as you can. I am now in my third year and so far, all is going well.

Renuka, third-year children's nursing field

Nicol (2019) argues that for learning to happen after receiving feedback, students need to make use of opportunities that are presented to them to enable them to construct their own meaning from the given feedback, to analyse it and make the suggested findings to further enhance future work both academically and clinically that will be assessed.

Students often view and interpret their feedback not at the task level, but rather more at a personal level (Kluger and DeNisi 1996). However, it is noted that although significant progress has been demonstrated in the quality of the assessment feedback being delivered, it remains one of the areas where students remain least satisfied with within higher education.

Addressing the lack of positive engagement from students with feedback is worrying for all, but under whose remit does it fall to actively encourage students to participate with feedback? The Higher Education Academy focus group found that the students expected the lecturers to lead on feedback and to be very explicit as to what and where exactly the focus needed to be (Winstone and Nash 2016).

In attempting to address this imbalance and disparity among student and lecturer, the Higher Education Academy developed the 'Developing Engagement with Feedback Toolkit' (DEFT) to support both parties to collaborate and work together in partnership. Designing the resources within the toolkit to be flexible means that aspects can be tailored and furnished to the individual student's needs.

Resources in the toolkit are presented in an easy, simple and logical fashion for the student to follow. They incorporate the use of flow-charts and additional information and ideas are on how to improve upon academic assignment writing. Clarity is provided as to what the purpose and function of feedback is and sets out standards and criteria for the same. DEFT acknowledges that feedback is and should be viewed as an additional learning resource. In efforts to further improve upon assessment feedback, lecturers and students should use and incorporate findings from other available resources, such as the Enhancing Assessment Feedback Practice in Higher Education: the EAT Framework (Evans 2020). The framework is underpinned by three principles:

1. Equity.
2. Agency.
3. Transparency.

One of the successes of the EAT framework is that it can be employed for students individually or for team working. In essence, the framework can be tailored to the learning needs of the student and/or team. This can help the student to increase not only their strengths but also help to further enhance weaker areas in a safe, controlled environment.

Complete this activity now

- Did you know that frameworks/toolkits such as the EAT framework existed?
- Do you think that they would be beneficial?
- Share with your colleagues what your views are on feedback and what improvements if any need to be amended.
- Do you feel that there is a difference in the quality of the feedback that you receive academically and that which you receive from your practice assessor and practice supervisors while in clinical placement?
- If yes, what do you think could be the reason?

Feedforward within the feedback process

Feedforward according to San Pedro (2012) allows the student to have the opportunity to make use of constructive advice offered in efforts to further improve upon and enhance future assignments. Hattie and Timperley (2007) state that feedforward is an essential and integral component of the whole feedback process (Figure 10.1). Providing feedback and feedforward has the potential to improve student outcomes. Improved student outcomes have the potential to improve patient care.

Wolstencroft and De Main (2020) found that the three-week or more turnaround period for marking commonplace within higher education in the UK may potentially contribute to perhaps the difficulties that students have in linking the advice offered to the submitted assignment, in

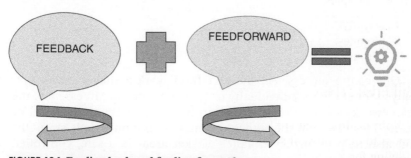

FIGURE 10.1 Feeding back and feeding forward.

TABLE 10.1	

Some methods related to electronic feedback.

Method	Description
Electronic publishing	With electronic publishing students can frequently refer to cumulative comments as they progress in the curriculum.
Audio capture	The use of digital recording provides an opportunity for those giving feedback to offer detailed feedback. This approach is particularly well suited to those who are auditory learners. Students can focus on and process comments when they choose, in the absence of their peers. Audio capture can be less ambiguous than feedback delivered verbally, face to face, and students can refer repeatedly to the feedback.
Visual and audio	This is also called screen casting; a video screen capture combines visual data and audio narration. A significant amount of engaging feedback can be given using screen casting, the student can save the feedback and then refer to it as needed. Screencasts capture the content on the computer screen while narrating
Blogs	Peer feedback can be given by blogs, which can improve student performance. Technology offers an ideal tool for expanding this approach. Blogs also encourage writing practice and facilitate peer feedback opportunities.

that within the period of marking they may have moved on from academic thinking to perhaps clinical placement.

There are other platforms that permit the delivery of feedforward. Technological advances were already being used and incorporated within higher education prior to the COVID-19 pandemic but, ultimately, over the past few years these advances have been somewhat accelerated and fast forwarded at a tremendous and often tumultuous pace.

Killingback et al. (2019) favour the use of technology; for example, podcasts to deliver feedforward with a particular focus and emphasis placed upon qualitative comments rather than just the mark awarded. See Table 10.1 for a discussion of some electronic feedback methods.

Simulated practice

Within healthcare there has always been designated simulated practice hours to develop skill sets and facilitate feedback, feedforward and debriefing for students. Ultimately, clinical simulation centres affiliated to higher education also had to embrace and adapt to the challenges that the COVID-19 pandemic has delivered. Innovative and creative learning platforms were introduced both for simulated practice and virtual placement.

Virtual reality placements and simulations not only offer up the opportunity to further enhance skill sets within a safe environment but in parallel with the lecturer feedback and debriefing, there is the opportunity for peer feedback and feedforward, which is invaluable (Bajaj et al. 2018; see also Chapters 3 and 5).

Alongside established simulation within healthcare, there has also been an increase in the use of virtual simulation within undergraduate nursing programmes. Foronda et al. (2018) suggest that virtual simulation is the platform for where previously simulation was carried out clinically, to be demonstrated and to participate with the learning on a virtual platform such as a computer, via the internet.

Nevertheless, despite all the innovative and creative approaches that have been introduced to facilitate continued learning, the development of an extensive armoury of skills, the facilitation of virtual placements to enable progression from one part of the programme to the next part, there must be student engagement. Without this the approaches will not successfully deliver on their preset (intended) learning outcomes. Of importance, it is noted that student engagement is crucial in determining and influencing both employability and professional development (Summers et al. 2013).

Over to you

- How do you feel taking part in simulated learning and being involved in virtual reality?
- What are your thoughts on giving peer feedback and feedforward to your colleagues?
- How do you feel when you are receiving peer feedback and feedforward from your colleagues?

Feedback via complaints and compliments

Complaints

Healthcare, as with any organisation, is only as good as its employees. Healthcare institutions strive constantly to deliver evidence-based practice that is seamless and safe for patients and their families, and many organisations incorporate these values and principles into their mission statement. A glance at social media outlets, of which there are many, can reveal a range of complaints, litigation, dissatisfaction with services, to mention but a few. How organisations maintain excellent standards of care delivery is complex. There are a range of internal processes and quality policies and procedures that must be adhered to.

Healthcare organisations are subjected to statutory regulation and scrutiny. They are responsible for and regulated to ensure that high quality care is provided. However, it should be remembered that we all have an important role to play in ensuring positive patient outcomes.

It is important to recognise that patients and their families have the right to complain about any aspect of their treatment and management while receiving NHS care and this decision to make concerns known is incorporated within the Department of Health and Social Care (2021). The NHS actively encourages feedback from patients, families and staff so that services can be improved upon.

Within the healthcare environment there is a designated team that advises patients and families on the process of making a complaint. In NHS settings, the advisors are known as the patient advice and liaison service often referred to as PALS. Private hospitals may have their own corporate route for raising concerns.

Service users, families and others can let the NHS know about their experience in one of two ways: provide feedback or make a complaint. There are two avenues that can be pursued if you wish to make a complaint. You can complain directly to the healthcare provider, for example the general practitioner, dental surgery or the hospital itself. Figure 10.2 highlights NHS England's complaints process.

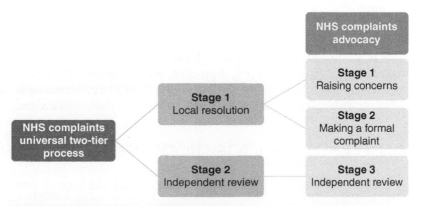

FIGURE 10.2 NHS England complaints process.

Some patients and their families may feel uncomfortable directly complaining to the healthcare provider. To ease the process, their complaint can be made directly to the commissioner of the service. Whichever route is explored, it is important to note that when making a complaint, it must be within 12 months of the incident or within 12 months of the matter coming to the attention of the person making the complaint.

NHS Resolution, previously the NHS Litigation Authority, manages negligence and other claims against the NHS in England on behalf of its member organisations. Its aim is in helping to resolve disputes fairly, sharing learning about risks and standards within the NHS and to help to improve safety for patients and staff. It is important to note, however, that anyone can complain or feedback about healthcare, its services and staff. If you have encountered unsafe practice, it is your duty to report the concern as you have a duty of care to ensure safety of patients. It should also be noted that complaints can be made against you, the student. The complaint would be structured around one of the four domains of the NMC Code of Professional Conduct (NMC 2018a):

- Prioritise people.
- Practice effectively.
- Preserve safety.
- Promote professionalism and trust.

Over to you

- Have you been involved in the complaint's procedure while on clinical placement?
- Have you witnessed unsafe practice, but felt uncomfortable to report it?

It is of paramount importance that if someone has complained about either your conduct or your clinical practice, you are furnished with the facts to enable you to appropriately respond. You should be presented with the facts in written format, and you will be requested to make a statement.

Some useful suggestions for you

- Make sure that you understand the what and the why of the complaint.

- Ensure that you are given a reasonable timeframe to prepare your statement.
- Keep your statement factual.
- Have clarity of what you did, saw, heard.
- Seek support from your academic assessor/academic guidance tutor.
- If you are a member of a union, please contact your representative.
- Do not submit your statement without it being reviewed.

Go online

Useful resources from the Royal College of Nursing to support and guide you with statement writing include:
- Statements: how to write them
- General statement template

www.rcn.org.uk/Get-Help/RCN-advice/statements

Depending on the nature of the complaint made, it could be followed up by a fitness to practise meeting. Fitness to practise is about managing the risk that a nurse poses to patients or members of the public in the future.

Go online

Advice regarding fitness to practice can be found in the NMC annual fitness to practise reports: www.nmc.org.uk/about-us/reports-and-accounts/fitness-to-practise-annual-report

You may have heard the term 'whistleblowing' with regard to an employee reporting wrongdoing within healthcare that they believe is in the public interest. An example of a whistleblower within healthcare is a doctor who raised concerns about mortality in the Bristol paediatric heart surgery scandal, which resulted in a public inquiry report in 2001.

An NHS nurse who was sacked after raising concerns regarding workloads contributing to a patient's death won her unfair dismissal case (BBC News 2020). Although difficult and distressing to report such concerns, these concerns were raised to promote the safety of their patients and, as such, both parties were acting as advocates for those patients within their care.

> ### Go online
>
> Nurses and all healthcare professionals have a duty of candour, the professional responsibility to be honest when things go wrong. A duty of candour requires nurses to be open and honest with patients but also to be open and honest within organisations in reporting adverse incidents or near misses that may have led to harm. The NMC has provided access to a webinar where you can find out more about the professional duty of candour and how to apply it in practice. You need to register to watch the webinar. Guidance on the professional duty of candour: www.nmc.org.uk/standards/guidance/the-professional-duty-of-candour
>
> There is also a series of slides that accompany the webinar, which you can download from the website page: Donohue, S. and Lewis, H. Professional Duty of Candour. 25 April 2022.

Clinical governance

Within most healthcare organisations, there is a culture of openness and transparency and the organisations adhere to clinical governance procedures. Clinical governance has been present for the past two to three decades and is instrumental in ensuring high standards of patient care. The introduction and subsequent implementation of clinical governance was as a direct result of whistleblowing concerns in Bristol.

NHS organisations must be accountable. They must ensure that there is provision in the workplace environments which enables the establishment and flourishment of excellence within clinical care (Scally and Donaldson 1998).

Also driving excellence within healthcare and minimising errors, near misses are quality metrics. The Agency for Healthcare Research and Quality discusses the Institute of Medicine (2001) and their identified six core domains that are critical in demonstrating quality healthcare is being delivered. All the core domains should be incorporated into all our daily practices within healthcare, no matter what clinical area or specialty that we are working in. We should all, when delivering care to patients ensure we are practising safe and effective person-centred care that encompasses the principles of being timely, equitable and efficient. Undoubtedly, this contributes to positive patient outcomes but also has an extremely crucial impact upon a healthcare organisation's quality rating and its position within the healthcare organisational league table.

Our attention thus far has focused upon the internal drivers, policies and procedures that are followed within healthcare. We now address the external regulated agencies that are pivotal in ensuring that the healthcare organisations are delivering safe and effective care alongside other quality metrics and indicators.

External regulated agencies

The Care Quality Commission (CQC) (2022) is an executive non-departmental public body of the Department of Health and Social Care in England. It was established in 2009 to regulate and inspect health and social care services in England. The CQC adheres to and ask the same five questions in all the healthcare organisational structures that they visit to measure safety and other criteria.

The basic premise of the inspection is to ensure safety for all; those who use services are protected from abuse and avoidable harm. Staff working within health and care organisations should be delivering effective care that is responsive to people's needs. Health and care organisations must demonstrate that they have appropriate infrastructures in place to keep people safe. An organisation cannot refuse inspection from the CQC or one of its equivalent bodies for other parts of the UK. Northern Ireland is regulated by the Regulation and Quality Improvement Authority, Wales by Care Inspectorate Wales, and Scotland by Care Inspectorate Scotland.

Members of the public can view the rating on the relevant organisation's website. The CQC publishes inspection reports on its website. This can prove useful and of benefit if a family wish to review residential and care homes for example, or indeed if you want to see the performance rating of your local healthcare organisation.

Go online

You may wish to review the CQC's rating and inspection reports of healthcare organisations to which you are going to be allocated: www. cqc.org.uk

Compliments

Within healthcare organisations, it is not just complaints that are received and are subsequently investigated; positive feedback is received also in the form of compliments. This can be received verbally from patients and family members, to written cards and letters arriving at the workplace after the patient has been discharged. The letters of compliment may come directly to the staff member in the clinical area, or the patient may send it to the chief executive or chief nurse of the organisation.

Write here

- Have you been complimented on your work performance by a patient and/or member of staff?

- How did you feel?

Although numerous handwritten cards and letters of compliments are sent yearly by patients and family members, Gillespie (2021) suggests that there is no standardised procedure for analysing these valuable data. Inevitably, the enriched positive feedback imparted within the letters of compliment is omitted from quality indicators and metrics within healthcare when measuring successful outcomes. Perhaps in the future this will be addressed, so that well-intentioned compliments can be incorporated with other data; for example, results from patient satisfaction surveys. However, you can ask your patient to record in your practice assessment document or e-practice assessment document (PAD/e-PAD) and, once registered, words of praise and compliments can be included in your revalidation documents (NMC 2021; see also Chapter 1).

Compliments are not only received from patients and family members but also from colleagues and peers. Nothing is as refreshing as either receiving compliments on an aspect of care that was delivered well or for you giving the positive compliment to another member of staff.

> ## Green flag
> Whenever you are having a challenging day in clinical placement, think back to when you received either a verbal or written compliment and how you felt. This can help to motivate you to get through the day.

Awards scheme

Undoubtedly, receiving compliments from patients and peers within your organisation is refreshing and valuable, and encourages you to keep being motivated and deliver excellent person-centred care, compliments can also be delivered via an awards scheme. Most healthcare organisations have in-house award ceremonies that staff can vote for the winners in each category. There is also a patient's award category. This is usually an annual event, and the nominees are recognised in a number of ways.

The Chief Nurse Awards (Chief Nurse Awards 2019) are another way of recognising excellence. There are two categories: the Silver Badge, for major contribution to patients and to the profession, and the Gold Medal, which recognises lifetime achievement for both nurses and midwives. Recipients are nominated by senior teams and report being overwhelmed to receive such an award and report continuing empowerment, determination and motivation.

Identifying and managing underperformance in student nurses: the action plan

As you progress throughout your education programme and move from one part to the next, your skill set, professionalism, critical thinking and judgement processes will be continually enhanced, in preparation for you to become a registrant on the NMC professional register. Contributing to all your clinical and professional development are your reflections of learning from others and professional feedback that are recorded within your PAD/e-PAD. Such enriched documentation demonstrates not only your knowledge and skills but your professionalism.

You will have heard not only from your lecturers but also from others the importance of having your documentation in your PAD/e-PAD completed and up to date (Chapter 9 discusses the PAD/e-PAD in more detail). This is of extreme importance when interviews are being carried out, assessing you against the set objectives agreed at initial interview, while you are on clinical placement.

Where there is appropriate, detailed feedback in your PAD/e-PAD, it can help, if necessary, in the early identification of underperformance, which ultimately will be of benefit to you and help you progress. This is why it is important that you ask your practice supervisors and practice assessor to document within your PAD/e-PAD in a timely manner.

As a student, you need to take ownership of your feedback. You need to be proactive in obtaining feedback on your performance. Negotiate a time early in your shift pattern that is convenient for you and your practice supervisor to meet to obtain feedback. Clinical environments are busy, so this can be challenging, but you still need to receive feedback. If you are working with the same supervisor for a few days, it would be acceptable for feedback to be entered at the end of those few days.

As you work predominantly with your practice supervisors, who are not only nurses but any member of the multidisciplinary team who is regulated by a professional body, it is important for your practice assessor that the relevant documentation is collated within your PAD/e-PAD for the interviews. If there is insufficient documentation within your PAD/e-PAD and concerns have been raised about areas of your practice or your professionalism, it makes for a very uneven platform to begin to discuss underperformance. By ensuring that you have completed, updated documentation in your PAD/e-PAD, this will enable a fair and equitable interview to be carried out by your practice assessor.

Try this on placement

- How difficult is it to receive feedback when on placement?
- In the care area are human factors always to blame when feedback is negative?
- Think about technological issues and how you might address them:
  - e-PAD not working
  - hospital firewall settings not allowing access
  - which device to use – mobile phone or laptop?
  - which web browser did you use?

If there are areas within your practice both clinically and professionally that need addressing and warrant the implementation of an action plan, allocated time needs to be set aside for the concerns to be discussed with you and actions agreed for helping you accomplish the new set objectives within an action plan. Your academic assessor will be invited to attend the meeting, so that you have support both clinically and academically.

Action plans generally seem to be viewed as a punishment or being punitive, whereas in reality they are structured, focused and initiated to establish goals by developing strategies to help you reach and achieve the goals. If an action plan is to be commenced, the lines of communication between you and your practice assessor and academic assessor have been fluid and that the concerns have been discussed with you. Guidance for raising concerns and the subsequent commencement of action plans can be found on the Pan London Practice Learning Group (2019) website. This is a useful resource for students.

Assessment of students is complex and staff need to be suitably prepared in the assessment process. The Standards for Student Supervision and Assessment (NMC 2018b) set out clear criteria on the different roles of both practice supervisor and practice assessor in the assessment process. They offer invaluable advice and resources for managing underperforming students and supporting the decision to not pass a student when in clinical practice. However, some practice assessors are failing to fail students within their clinical areas. Duffy (2003), in the seminal work on failing to fail, highlights and offers suggestions as to why this is occurring. Perhaps assessors are lacking in confidence despite receiving preparation. Clinical placement areas are extremely busy, and there may be an unwillingness to invest the time required to fail a student, added to this the emotional impact of not passing a student.

A supervisor's notes

Recently, working with a practice assessor, we had to fail a second-year nursing student, and I can tell you, this was one of the most taxing things I have had to do in my nursing career.

I pride myself on my high standards and I think I am fair when it comes to working with students and discussing their performance with them and the practice assessor. I offer students lots of support as they work towards achieving their competencies but, the student in question was unable to demonstrate that she was competent in a number of areas.

Allowing a student who does not meet fitness for practice standards to progress, I think is a significant concern. I also think it could be seen as a breach of ethical responsibility and professional accountability.

The practice assessor, myself, the student and the academic assessor put together an action plan for the student to be able to demonstrate competence. We worked in a transparent and objective way to support the student who eventually passed the outstanding competencies.

It was a really difficult time for all of us, but we worked together, and we all supported each other; it was so pleasing to see a positive outcome. Failing a student in practice has an impact on all members of the team but, our key aim was to offer support.

The student has asked if she can come back to our ward to do her management placement and of course we are delighted to have her back.

Mei Mei, staff nurse oncology ward

An action plan can be put in place for any concerns relating to practice and your professionalism. Examples of what could be included in a plan are punctuality issues, time management and prioritisation of care. An example of an action plan will be discussed later.

Complete this activity now

- Have you heard of action plans?
- For what reasons do you think you can be put on an action plan?
- Have you been required to work on an action plan?
- If so, did you think that it was fair?
- How do you think your practice assessor feels discussing concerns with you, and placing you on an action plan?

Regardless of the location of your clinical placement, action plans should be standardised and should follow a similar format. An action plan can be commenced at any time of your placement, even on your last day. Once the area(s) of concern has been identified and discussed with you in an open, transparent forum where the opportunity to actively contribute to the discussion and state your own views on whether you agree with the concerns, the plan is drawn up and immediately instigated.

The action plan must incorporate SMART (specific, measurable, achievable, realistic, timebound) objectives. Using the SMART objectives affords for structured learning,(see also Chapter 11). In addition, it provides focus and motivation to enable you to progress. Within the plan, there will be clarity on what the expectations are, what are the priorities and tasks to be achieved. A clear timeline will also be included in the plan, and that the plan will be constantly monitored and evaluated with an agreed weekly review meeting between you and your practice assessor. If the action plan is not passed, it gets carried forward to your next placement. Table 10.2 provides an example of an action plan.

Action plans must be agreed, signed and dated by you the student and also by both your practice and academic assessors. The placement name and date that the plan was commenced must also be recorded within the action plan.

In the action plan of 'Prioritise People' (Table 10.2), the measures of success have been broken down into weekly components and then increased if improvement has been demonstrated. This is to give the student time to build upon their confidence levels and improve their skill set, while maintaining patient safety which is essential.

By working to an action plan, will help the student to focus upon the areas that need improvement. The support of both the practice and academic assessors will be available and if a member of a nursing union (Royal College of Nursing or Unison) support can also be accessed here, as well as the National Union of Students. Some students are upset and feel sad at being placed on a plan, whereas others welcome the plan to help them to develop clinically and professionally.

While working to achieve the components of an action plan, the student will usually work with the same staff member(s) so that consistency can be witnessed as the student progresses through the plan. Weekly meetings should be arranged with the practice assessor to enable review of the plan and to document improvements or any cause for concern.

Following the weekly review, the practice assessor can pass the student on some of the components of the action plan if they have been achieved, but consistency needs to be demonstrated and the plan, if it is to be passed, is usually signed off at the same time of as the final interview within the placement area.

Not all plans are successfully achieved, however, and will need to be carried forward to the next placement area. This will be clearly documented within the PAD/e-PAD so that the next practice assessor is aware that a plan is in existence. If the plan has not been passed in the final placement of year three, the student will have to carry out a retrieval placement to complete the action plan.

TABLE 10.2

An example of an action plan.

Nature of concern (refer to professional value(s), and/or episode of care)	What does the student need to demonstrate? Objectives and measures of success (measurable, achievable and realistic)	Support available	Date for review (timed)	Review/ feedback
1: Prioritise people: Student Nurse Arthur Ward (third year) is not demonstrating that he can prioritise people and his workload effectively and safely.	1: Student Nurse Arthur Ward to demonstrate in the remaining weeks of this placement (4) safe and effective prioritisation of patients in his care. **Week one:** Student will care for only two patients per shift, plan care for the patients and discuss this plan with nurse that he is working alongside. Student must always work within scope of practice. **Week two:** Student to increase patient case load to three if has been successful in demonstrating improvement in prioritising people and workload in week one. **Week three and four:** Student to be safely and effectively planning and prioritising care for four patients in his care daily.	**Practice assessor: Name:** Jane Roberts **Academic assessor: Name:** Robert Gere	**Weekly review. 1st review:** 09/02/2022 **2nd review:** 16/02/2022 **3rd review:** 23/02/2022 **4th review:** 02/03/2022 – to coincide with final interview	**Date: Comments:** Weekly comments following review on any signs of improvements or any other concerns, following discussion with the student. **Practice assessor: Name:** Jane Roberts **Signature:**
Student name: Arthur Ward Practice assessor name: Jane Roberts Academic assessor name: Robert Gere	Student signature: *Arthur Ward* Practice assessor signature: *Jane Roberts* Academic assessor signature: *Robert Gere*	Date: 02/02/2022 Date: 02/02/2022 Date: 02/02/2022	Placement name: Mandela Ward	Date action plan initiated: 02/02/2022

Summary

This chapter has focused on feedback and feedforward and how the student should be actively involved in receiving both from practice assessors, supervisors and the team of lecturers. Engagement with assessors is essential for a student to develop academically and clinically throughout the programme of study.

Regulatory bodies and their inspection processes have been discussed, together with the NHS complaints procedure, which aim to improve upon existing services within health and care organisations and ultimately ensure patient safety.

Finally, action plans have been discussed, and the difficulties that practice assessors have when concerned with underperformance, and why some find failing a student difficult. Discussion has centred upon the importance of ensuring that students work within their professional scope of practice to keep patients safe while they are in health and care organisations.

References

Agency for Healthcare Research and Quality (2001). *Six Domains of Healtcare Quality*. www.ahrq.gov/talkingquality/measures/six-domains.html (accessed 18 March 2023).

Bajaj, K., Meguerdichian, M., Thoma, B. et al. (2018). The PEARLS Healthcare Debriefing Tool. *Academic Medicine* 93 (2): 336. https://doi.org/10.1097/ACM.0000000000002035.

BBC News (2020). *Hartlepool NHS whistleblower nurse wins dismissal case*. BBC News, 4 March. https://www.bbc.co.uk/news/uk-england-tees-51728490 (accessed 18 March 2023).

Care Quality Commission (2022). *The Five Key Questions We Ask*. www.cqc.org.uk/what-we-do/how-we-do-our-job/five-key-questions-we-ask (accessed August 2022).

Department of Health and Social Care (2021). *NHS Complaints Guidance*. www.gov.uk/government/publications/the-nhs-constitution-for-england/how-do-i-give-feedback-or-make-a-complaint-about-an-nhs-service (accesses 18 March 2023).

Duffy, K. (2003). *Failing Students: A qualitative study of factors that influence the decisions regarding assessment of students' competence in practice*. Glasgow: Caledonian Nursing and Midwifery Research Centre.

Evans, C. (2020). *EAT Framework*. www.eatframework.com (accessed 18 March 2023).

Foronda, C.L., Swobodsa, S.M., Henry, M.N. et al. (2018). Student preferences and perceptions of learning from VSim for nursing. *Nurse Education Practice* 33: 27–32.

Gibbs, G. and Simpson, C. (2004). Conditions under which assessment supports students' learning. *Learning and Teaching in Higher Education* 1 (1): 3–31.

Gillespie, A. (2021). Identifying and encouraging high-quality healthcare: an analysis of the content and aims of patient letters of compliment. *BMJ Quality and Safety* 30: 484–492.

Hattie, J. and Timperley, H. (2007). The power of feedback. *Review of Educational Research* 83: 70–120.

Institute for Academic Development (2016). *Feedback: Quick Ideas*. University of Edinburgh. www.ed.ac.uk/institute-academic-development/learning-teaching/staff/assessment/quick-ideas (accessed 18 March 2023).

Jessop, T. (2019). Changing the narrative. In: *Innovative Assessment in Higher Education: A Handbook for Academic Practitioners* (ed. C. Bryan and K. Clegg), 36–49. Abingdon: Routledge.

Johnson, A. (2013). Facilitating productive use of feedback in higher education. *Active Learning in Higher Education* 14: 63–76.

Killingback, C., Ahmed, O., and Williams, J. (2019). 'It was all in your voice.' Tertiary student perceptions of alternative feedback modes (audio, video, podcast, and screencast): a qualitative literature review. *Nurse Education Today* 72: 32–39. https://doi.org/10.1016/j.nedt.2018.10.012.

King, D. (2022). The use of online formative assessment and the impact on student performance. *Irish Journal of Academic Practice* 10 (1552): 7. https://doi.org/10.21427/cxd5-dz42.

Kluger, A.N. and DeNisi, A. (1996). The effects of feedback interventions on performance. A historical review, a meta-analysis, and a preliminary feedback intervention theory. *Psychological Bulletin* 119: 254–284.

Mc Callum, S. and Milner, M. (2021). The effectiveness of formative assessment: student views and staff reflections. *Assessment and Evaluation in Higher Education* 46 (1): 1–16. https://doi.org/10.1080/02602938.2020.1754761.

NHS England (2019). *Chief Nursing Officer for England and Chief Midwifery Officer Awards*. www.england.nhs.uk/nursingmidwifery/chief-nursing-officer-for-england (accessed 18 March 2023).

Nicol, D. (2019). The power of internal feedback: exploiting natural comparison processes. *Assessment and Evaluation in Higher Education* 46 (5): 756–778. https://doi.org/10.1080/02602938.2020.1823314.

Nursing and Midwifery Council (2018a). *The Code: Professional standards of practice and behaviour for nurses, midwives and nursing associates.* www.nmc.org.uk/standards/code (accessed 18 March 2023).

Nursing and Midwifery Council (2018b). *Realising Professionalism: Standards for Education and Training. Part 2: Standards for Student Supervision and Assessment.* www.nmc.org.uk/Student-supervision-assessment (accessed 18 March 2023).

Nursing and Midwifery Council (2021). *Revalidation.* www.nmc.org.uk/revalidation (accessed 18 March 2023).

Pan London Practice Learning Group (2019). *Raising Concerns Facilitators Guide.* https://plplg.uk/sssa-resources (acessed 18 March 2023).

Pokorny, H. (2021). Assessment for learning. In: *Enhancing Learning Through Assessment* (ed. H. Pokorny and D. Warren), 79–105. Newbury Park, CA: Sage.

Pokorny, H. and Pickford, P. (2010). Complexity, cues and relationships in student feedback. *Active Learning in Higher Education* 11 (1): 21–29.

Sambell, K., McDowell, L., and Montgomery, C. (2012). *Assessment for Learning in Higher Education*. Abingdon: Routledge.

San Pedro, M. (2012). Feedback and feedforward: focal points for improving academic performance. *Journal of Technology and Science Education* 2 (2): 77–85.

Scally, G. and Donaldson, L.J. (1998). Clinical governance and the drive for quality improvement in the new NIIS in England. *British Medical Journal* 317 (7150): 61–65.

Summers, P., Pearson, D., Gough, S., and Siekierski, J. (2013). The effects on student engagement of employing students in professional roles. In: *Student Engagement: Identity, Motivation and Community* (ed. C. Nygaard, S. Brand, P. Bartholomew, and L. Millard), 35–54. Faringdon: Libri.

Winstone, N. and Nash, R. (2016). *The Developing Engagement with Feedback Toolkit (DEFT)*. York: Higher Education Academy. https://www.advance-he.ac.uk/knowledge-hub-developing-engagement-feedback-toolkit-deft (accessed 19 March 2023).

Wolstencroft, P. and De Main, L. (2020), 'Why didn't you tell me that before?' Engaging undergraduate students in feedback and feedforward within UK higher education. *Journal of Further and Higher Education* 45 (3): 312–323. https://doi.org/10.1080/030 w9877X.2020.1759517.

CHAPTER 11

The student as a teacher

Ashley Luchmun

AIM

This chapter explores the role of the student nurse/trainee nursing associate as a teacher and facilitator of peers in learning.

LEARNING OUTCOMES

Having read this chapter, the reader will:

1. Understand the context of the student nurse/trainee nursing associate as a teacher.
2. Explore the responsibilities as teacher and facilitator of learning.
3. Make links between the role of teacher and the Nursing and Midwifery Council (NMC) Code (NMC 2018c).
4. Identify appropriate methods of teaching.
5. Understand the responsibilities of delegation.

Succeeding on your Nursing Placement: Supervision, Learning and Assessment for Nursing Students, First Edition. Edited by Ian Peate.
© 2024 John Wiley & Sons Ltd. Published 2024 by John Wiley & Sons Ltd.

Introduction

As part of their learning journey, the learner will have some teaching responsibilities as well as delegation decisions to make. It might seem strange that you are currently enrolled as a student nurse or trainee nursing associate and yet there will be an expectation that you will be teaching others. Nurse education is different from childhood and younger ages education as there is an emphasis on the adult learning nature of the process. Adult learning can be described as a lifelong process which can present challenges in defining. Adult learning consists of distinct aspects: assimilation of knowledge, skills and attitudes (Abela 2009). Values can also be added to this list as they are part of the NMC Standards of Education (NMC 2018a,b,c,d, 2022) and universally qualified as a requirement for students as well as registrants. The University and College Union (2009) adds that there is an emphasis on learning as active transmission of knowledge and skills. The NMC (2018d) additionally states that education for nurses providing general care needs to include 'the ability to participate in the practical training of health personnel'.

Peer learning has been around for a long while; more experienced students provide peer mentoring, where they mentor, educate and act as role models to their less experienced peers (Jacobsen et al. 2022). The NMC (2018d) standards emphasises peer teaching and learning. Student nurses in their final year of the programme are required to have an episode of care whereby they 'will be given the opportunity to supervise and teach a junior learner/colleague in practice and provide a written reflection on this experience' (NMC 2018d). Having a learning culture forms part of the standards of education and this starts in the nurse education programme and carries on way past qualification and registration (NMC 2018a).

The student teacher and the Nursing and Midwifery Council

The ability to teach and support others is not an optional skill but is a requirement as stipulated by section 4.1 of the standards of proficiency for registered nurses (NMC 2018a, p. 30). This section states that registered nurses need to 'demonstrate effective supervision, teaching and performance appraisal'. A student nurse especially at the end of their programme should be able to supervise and teach less experienced students and junior colleagues. Trainee nursing associates are also required to teach and supervise according to their level of competence. What does supervising, learning, and teaching mean?

Write here

Before moving on to the next section, what is you understanding of supervising and teaching?

Supervising:

Teaching:

Supervising and teaching

There are fundamental differences between supervision known as clinical supervision and supervising; understanding the terminology is essential to avoid misunderstanding. Clinical supervision has been described as protected time where learners and practitioners can reflect on their practice to improve the quality of their care (Bond and Holland 2011, Saab et al. 2021). While clinical supervision has its value in teaching and learning, it is not a main subject for this chapter, but will form part of learning as both student and eventually health practitioner.

Teaching from the perspective of the student nurse or trainee nursing associate can be simplistically described as the facilitation of learning for peers, as well as other members of the multidisciplinary team (MDT). If we explore further, we can also agree that it is the ability to impart knowledge and skills, as well as values and attitudes, which can then arguably be categorised as professional nursing beliefs.

Box 11.1 | Andragogy and pedagogy

Before venturing further into theory, it is relevant to explore two major education concepts. As mentioned at the beginning of this chapter, nurse education is adult education and therefore the teaching strategies will be different to other types of education.

Pedagogy in its simplistic definition means the art and science of teaching children (Knowles 1980). Pedagogy is further expanded as including learning, teaching and development, influenced by cultural, social and political values and principles (Education Scotland 2005). Knowles (1980) clarifies that pedagogy might present challenges for adult education which leads for arguments for andragogy.

Andragogy in its simplistic definition places more focus on the adult learner as an independent entity who needs to understand the reasons behind the learning. This then becomes more self-directed (Knowles 1980; Rachal 2002; Pew 2007; Noor et al. 2012).

Before discussing the role of the student as a teacher further, it is worthwhile to explore briefly some the most common theories of learning and teaching. Box 11.1 differentiates andragogy and pedagogy.

Learning

Theories of learning: a brief listing

Understanding learning can make teaching more effective. Before proceeding further, it is helpful to make the difference between *learning* and *teaching*. These two terms are often used in the same sentence and can create the impression that they have the same meaning.

Learning tends to be more internal, with the learner's personal cognitive qualities influencing it, whereas *teaching* is the act of facilitating the learning either formally (with the use of didactic methods of teaching) or informally (such as role modelling, reflection and observation). Prozescky (2000) cautions with the perception of teaching as most of us perceive teaching as what we ourselves have experienced as learners. This gets more interesting when we consider the teacher as a learner which links well with reflective practice in teaching (Maynard et al. 2016). Seven influential theories of learning are identified (Table 11.1)

Over to you

Before moving on to the next section, spend some time reflecting on the above learning theories and write a few sentences describing your own learning methods. Think about when you think you learn better and probably still remember the learning achieved even now.

TABLE 11.1

Most influential theories of learning.

Behaviourist theories	These suggest that learning happens in response to stimuli. The performance is then improved through a reward system and reinforced through exercise and repetition. Methods of instruction are then step by step approaches where the learner gets assessed and rewarded especially for 'correct' behaviour.
Cognitive psychology	Learning is seen as the acquisition of knowledge. The learner then becomes a receiver of information and must process and store this in their memory. Methods of instruction are lecturing and reading textbooks and articles (similar to what it is that you are doing here).
Constructivism	Learners are not seen as passive receivers of information and knowledge. Learners are supported to make sense of the information on their own and there is an emphasis on interpreting the knowledge. Methods of instruction would be facilitating the learner to develop their own learning objectives based on their needs.
Social constructivism	This was put forward by Albert Bandura (Bandura 1977), who describes cognitive and behavioural frameworks and encompasses theories of motivation and attention. This theory of learning suggests that people learn within a social context, and that learning is facilitated through concepts such as role-modelling, observational learning, and imitation. Methods of instruction from the student nurse/trainee nursing associate perspective as a teacher would be encouraging junior learners to learn from observation of good practice.

(*Continued*)

TABLE **11.1**	
(Continued)	
Experiential learning	Experiential learning theories build on social and constructivist theories of learning. It suggests that learners learn by practising. Carl Rogers (Rogers 1951) suggested that learning should be self-initiated, and that learning can be facilitated and not be done directly.
Multiple intelligences	Howard Gardner (Gardner 2000) proposes that we all learn in our own unique specific way. The teacher therefore needs to recognise that their learners will have different ways of learning, and this will need to be considered when designing teaching activities.
Situated learning theory and community of practice	According to the theory, it is within communities that learning occurs most effectively. Interactions taking place within a community of practice (CoP). CoP's are groups of people who share a common concern, a set of problems, or an interest in a topic They need to come together to support individual and group goals.

Source: Adapted from International Bureau of Education (2022).

Theories of teaching

Now that you have been briefly introduced to learning theories, it is relevant to investigate teaching theories. From simple association, we can agree that theories of teaching would be influenced by those of learning. Dewey (1984) made the analogy that teaching is to learning as selling is to buying.

A teacher should be able to convince the learner that what they are being taught is relevant and has value and this can then lead to a change of behaviour(s). Rajagopalan (2019) goes further and describes teaching as a 'scientific process, and its major components are content, communication and feedback'. There is general agreement that teaching is a process rather than a one-off activity. For teaching to be more effective having a structured approach is essential.

Approaches to teaching

For teaching to be a process, having a structured approach will be helpful. Figure 11.1 illustrates how teaching planning can be simplistically interpreted as a three-way approach. At the beginning of the cycle, we

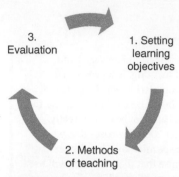

FIGURE 11.1 **Simple approach to teaching planning.**

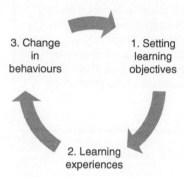

FIGURE 11.2 **Adapted approach to teaching planning.**

have the identification of learning objectives, which then lead to deciding what teaching methods can be used and ends with an evaluation of the learning. This can be adapted further with the methods associated with learning experiences, especially if multiple intelligences are to be considered (Figure 11.2). The methodology would therefore be adapted to the learning needs of the learner with the evaluation being the change in behaviour(s) in both the short and the long term.

Learning objectives

As discussed in chapter 9 regarding the practice assessment document, you will normally set up your learning objectives prior to or at the beginning of starting a placement. This setting of objectives needs to a planned process with your practice assessors and practice supervisors. Mohanna et al. (2011) identify four steps in an educational cycle:

1. Assessment of learning needs.
2. Setting objectives.
3. Choosing methods of teaching.
4. Evaluating learning.

Assessment of learning needs

As a student, no matter what year of study, you are in, you will be a role model to other students and trainees, and you will also be representing the profession. To make learning meaningful, it is necessary to identify the learning needs. Different individuals will have varying learning needs. You might be informally or formally approached by other students to either support or teach them. This could happen at any stage of your programme of study. In the final year, for example, you are required as a student nurse or trainee nursing associate to 'supervise and teach a junior learner/colleague in practice'. This will constitute one of the two episodes of care you will need to achieve before you complete your clinical placements in the final year (Box 11.2).

Box 11.2 | Learning outcomes for episodes of care

Pre-registration nursing students in year 3

1. Supervise and teach less experienced students and colleagues, appraising the quality of the nursing care they provide, documenting performance, promoting reflection, and providing constructive feedback.
2. Demonstrate an understanding of the factors that both facilitate and impede learning in practice.
3. Demonstrate leadership potential in the assessment, planning, implementation and evaluation of care.
4. Apply the appropriate knowledge and skills in appraising the quality of the nursing care provided by the junior learner colleague.
5. Demonstrate effective verbal/non-verbal communication and interpersonal skills in engaging with the learner and others involved in the care and act as a positive role model.

6. Critically reflect on their own role and the role of the nurse in the supervision, facilitation and evaluation of learning for the whole team.

Trainee nursing associates in year 2

1. Support, supervise and act as a role model to nursing associate students, health care support workers and those new to care roles, reviewing the quality of care they provide, promoting reflection and providing constructive feedback.

2. Demonstrate an ability to support and motivate junior learner colleagues, other members of the care team and interact confidently with them.

3. Demonstrate the ability to monitor and review the quality of care delivered by the junior learner colleague providing clear constructive feedback.

4. Demonstrate effective verbal, non-verbal communication, and interpersonal skills in engaging with the junior learner and others involved in the care giving clear instructions and explanations during supervision.

5. Reflect on their own role and the role of the junior learner colleague in the supervision encouraging the learner to reflect on their practice.

Source: Adapted from Practice Learning Group (2021).

Maintaining boundaries is recommended if you will be formally teaching and evaluating a peer. It is necessary to have a formal meeting with your learner and discuss what their learning needs are, and this meeting is an ideal opportunity to clarify roles which helps with the setting of boundaries. At this stage of your learning journey, it would be advisable for you to choose only one specific area where you can teach a peer.

Identifying learning needs works better if the learner self-identifies the gaps in their knowledge. However, sometimes, you as the teacher need to act as a facilitator to help the learner identify these needs. You would have the advantage of having been in a possibly similar situation when you were in year 1. However, a word of warning would be not to avoid assuming that the learner would have the same learning needs as yourself. Please be aware of self-fulfilling prophecies, as each learner is different and their needs will be different. Box 11.3 gives some tips to avoid self-fulfilling prophecies.

Green flag

Self-fulfilling prophecies are instances where expectations or percep-tions (mostly false or incorrect) lead to the expectations or perceptions becoming true. In teaching situations, a self-fulfilling prophecy can oc-cur if the teacher holds initially incorrect expectations about a student and the resulting social interaction leads to the student to behave in such a manner to confirm the expectation.

Box 11.3 | Tips to avoid self-fulfilling prophecies

- Support peers to think about their thinking.
- Advise on completing SWOT (strengths, weaknesses, opportunities, threats) analysis.
- Flip roles – put yourself in the role of the student (explore feelings and anxieties)
- Communicate clearly and honestly.
- Give constructive and honest feedback.
- Give formative feedback.
- Set achievable objectives.

Setting learning objectives

Once the learning needs are identified, these might be vague and mostly conceptual. For example, your learner might want to learn more about wound care, which will be relevant for the nursing course but wound care on its own is a wide topic so this needs to be narrowed down further. Setting SMART objectives is key in increasing the chances of success.

SMART objectives SMART is an acronym for helping with the writing of learning objectives and can also be used for other goals setting frame-works (Table 11.2). Using the SMART framework can help with writing meaningful learning objectives.

Identifying an appropriate action verb in setting SMART objectives is a vital part for both the learner and teacher. For the learner, this is

TABLE 11.2				
The SMART acronym.				
S	**M**	**A**	**R**	**T**
Specific learning objectives	Measurable learning objectives	Achievable learning objectives	Relevant learning objectives	Time bound learning objectives
The learning objective (LO) should be clear and well-defined. Avoid the use of complex or vague terminology if possible and the LO should have the same meaning for both learner and teacher. Setting an appropriate action verb is also essential and this will be addressed in the next section. Examples of specific LO: *Complete a Waterlow score Complete a NEWS2 chart.*	Measurable The LO should be measurable, that is, the teacher should be able to measure the success of what is the desired target. Here are some examples of measurable LOs: *Complete a Waterlow score accurately Complete a NEWS2 chart accurately.*	Achievable The LO should be achievable in the agreed time frame. The teacher needs to consider any prior knowledge the learner has. The examples cited will work but will only be achievable if the learner has existing knowledge of the assessment tools (Waterlow and NEWS2).	The LO must be meaningful to the learning needs and in the context of the examples, the learner must know when to complete and the context of the risk assessments.	The LO needs to have a time frame for achievement. Having timeframes helps the learner sets noticeable urgency to achieve the target.

important as it makes the learning objectives clearer and facilitates the ability to measure their success at attainment. For the teacher, it helps to structure the teaching methodologies appropriately. *Taxonomy* is a term that can be used to describe the classification of themes. In the context of education, a taxonomy can serve to design and structure learning goals and objectives (Tuma and Nassar 2021). The most common taxonomies are:

- Structure of the observed learning outcome (SOLO) taxonomy (Box 11.4; (Biggs and Collis 1982).
- The six facets of understanding (Box 11.5; Wiggins and McTighe 2005).
- Educational objectives (Box 11.6; Bloom 1956).
- Taxonomy of significant learning (Box 11.7; Fink 2003).

Box 11.4 | Structure of the Observed Learning Outcome (SOLO) Taxonomy

- Prestructural – learner knows nothing about the topic.
- Unistructural – learner understands one or two elements. Verb examples: memorise, identify, define
- Multistructural – learner has acquired knowledge and can use it.
  Verb examples: classify, describe, discuss, select, outline
- Relational – learner has deeper understanding and demonstrates complex thinking.
  Verbs examples: apply, integrate, analyse, predict, conclude, summarise
- Extended abstract – learner has sophisticated understanding and can apply this in different circumstances.
  Verbs examples: theorise, reflect, generate, create, hypothesise

Source: Adapted from Biggs and Collis (1982).

Box 11.5 | Six facets of understanding

- Explanation – learners explain or justify their course of action.
  Verbs examples: demonstrate, describe, read, write, teach, justify
- Interpretation – learners can make sense of information.
  Verb examples: critique, evaluate, investigate, illustrate

- Application – learners put knowledge in context and apply to practice.
  Verb examples: adapt, connect, create, design, produce, solve
- Perspective – learners can see other views and take a critical stance.
  Verb examples: analyse, argue, compare, debate, infer
- Empathy – learners demonstrate intellectual imagination.
  Verb examples: be open to, believe, consider, debate, relate
- Self-knowledge – learners can understand their own progress and understanding.
  Verb examples: realise, be aware of, reflect, recognise, self-assess

Source: Wiggins and McTighe (2005).

Box 11.6 | Bloom's taxonomy

Educational objectives

Bloom taxonomy is a well-known structure still used today in designing educational programmes. While it has its critics and has been revised on many occasions by other theorists, it is still very popular. Bloom's taxonomy identifies six levels of cognitive domains and complexity. From these domains, the action verbs are then derived.

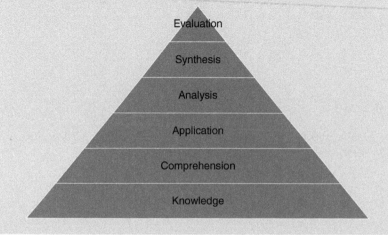

Evaluation

Synthesis

Analysis

Application

Comprehension

Knowledge

- Knowledge – recalling facts and information.
  Verb examples: arrange, define, label, list, memorise
- Comprehension – able to explain ideas and concepts.
  Verb examples: classify, describe, explain, recognise
- Application – use learnt information in new situations.
  Verb examples: apply, choose, demonstrate, solve
- Analysis – make connections between ideas and concepts.
  Verb examples: analyse, appraise, categorise, compare
- Synthesis – putting ideas and understanding together to
  form a whole.
  Verb examples: arrange, assemble, design, formulate
- Evaluation – judgement on existing knowledge and creation
  of new concepts.
  Verb examples: assess, estimate, judge, evaluate

Source: Adapted from Bloom (1956).

Box 11.7 | Fink's taxonomy

- Fink argues that active learning through experiential learning
  can be more valuable and adds that learning is interactive
  and different types of learning can influence each other. Six
  aspects of learning are identified in Fink's taxonomy.

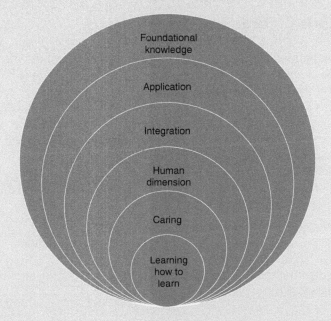

- Foundational knowledge – this is the stage where the learner acquires and remembers information and ideas.
  Verb examples: identify, explain, indicate, list
- Application – this aspect involves critical, creative, and practical thinking.
  Verb examples: analyse, assess, critique, demonstrate
- Integration – this involves making connections between different concepts and can also include experiential knowledge.
  Verb examples: Blend, connect, compare, contrast
- Human dimension – this is where learners learn more about themselves but also about others who they interact with.
  Verb examples: acquire, advise, advocate, behave
- Caring – learners care more about what they are learning which makes the learning more meaningful.
  Verb examples: develop, discover, explore, identify
- Learning how to learn – this is where learners understand their own learning and engage in self-directed learning. This then supports life-long learning.
  Verb examples: reflect, research, self-assess, self-regulate

Source: Adapted from Fink (2003).

Methods of teaching and learning

Having identified learning needs and learning objectives, the next step would be choosing and identifying teaching methods. There is no ideal method of teaching but rather appropriate ones. It is essential to remember at this stage to also highlight the 'new learner' in the relative high technology influence in health care education (Bezanilla et al. 2019). Several teaching methodologies can be identified (Box 11.8). It will be up to the teacher to decide which method is more appropriate; sometimes a combination of methodologies can be used.

Bezanilla et al. (2019) also identifies three main aspects of methodologies of teaching; these are:

1. Oral and written methodologies.
2. Active methodologies, such as case studies and collaborative learning.
3. Other methodologies, such as follow-up, questioning and flipped classrooms.

Box 11.8 | Teaching methods

Teacher centred:
- Lecture
- Explanation
- Instruction
- Story telling

Interaction between teacher and learner:
- Conversation
- Discussion
- Demonstration
- Modelling
- Problem solving

Learner centred:
- Reflection
- Brainstorming/mind mapping
- Self-directed learning
- Teacher provides feedback

Source: Adapted from Landøy et al. (2019).

For your context in facilitating and supporting a junior student or colleague, three main methods of teaching will be helpful:

1. Role modelling.
2. Opportunistic teaching.
3. Teaching practical skills.

This list is not exhaustive but these are the most likely opportunities and are now discussed.

Role modelling The NMC (2018a) states that registered nurses need to act as role-models. This can also be seen as a method of teaching as demonstration of good practice can engender good practice learning as student learning is influenced by the behaviour of professionals in clinical practice (Baldwin et al. 2014). Bandura (1977) described social interaction as a way of learning. Students learn and are influenced by observing others and the degree by which this is successful depends on (Murray and Main 2005):

- The development of a professional relationship between the learner and the teacher.

- The relevance and usefulness of what is being modelled (linked to the learning objectives).
- The learner's ability to complete the task.
- The learner's motivation.

Attributes of positive role-modelling Role-modelling can be both positive (demonstrating good practice) and negative (demonstrating not so good practice). Both can lead to learning. It is important to point out that negative role-modelling can also lead to learning in terms of 'what not to do' (in case of observing what not to do, please refer to your institution raising concerns policies). Box 11.9 lists several possible positive role-modelling attributes and traits.

Green flag

You were (or are) a first-year student or trainee; think about all the positive role modelling you have come across. Think about how you can replicate and demonstrate good practice in your journey. Try to remember these roles models and those attributes that made them good role models.

Box 11.9 | Positive role-modelling attributes and traits

- Be genuinely interested
- Show empathy for learners
- Be positive
- Punctuality
- Honesty
- Integrity
- Show willingness to teach
- Ensure confidentiality
- Show respect
- Enthusiasm to teaching
- Be caring and supportive
- Give constructive feedback
- Be patient
- Promote evidence-based health care

Motivation

Hear it from the student

I was on clinical placement with a district nursing team, with two other students (one a student nurse and one a trainee nursing associate) including Raj. We are both students at the same university. I am in the same cohort as Raj, but I don't know him as he is in a different group. On the first few days of placement, I tried to engage in conversation with Raj but, although he is polite, he doesn't seem to be too keen to engage in conversation me. He appears very quiet and aloof. During the next few weeks, Raj appeared disinterested in team handovers, and he doesn't seem interested in teaching sessions either. He is regularly seen on his mobile phone texting. Raj has been told by his practice assessor that he needs to be more pro-active and needs to seek out learning opportunities. Despite the several prompts, Raj has not been able to have similar outreach learning opportunities as I have. He has had low attendance at placement and has also been late on a couple of shifts.

Arturo, first year mental health nurse

Over to you

- What do you think could be happening?
- How can these issues be addressed?
- How can Raj be supported?

Motivation is essential in all learning activities but can be subject to variation and depends upon the learning environment. When motivation starts decreasing, this can impact negatively on the effectiveness of both teaching and learning (Murphy 2006).

Motivation has two main aspects: positive and negative motivation. Positive motivation will be where the learner is keen to learn new skills or develop themselves and therefore will be more likely to succeed in achieving their goals. In negative motivation, the learner will have fears of failure or not passing an assessment, for example, and this can motivate them to perform better. However, positive motivation tends to lead to better long-term learning outcomes (Bye et al. 2007; Mohanna et al. 2011).

Ryan and Deci (2000) further identify intrinsic and extrinsic motivational factors, which are relevant. Intrinsic factors tend to be positive motivation while extrinsic tend to be negative motivation although this is obviously not always the case. Ryan and Deci (2000) further identify three aspects of motivation:

1. Autonomy – this is where the learner has some control over their actions, and this can be influenced by prior learning and experience.
2. Competence – this is where the learner needs to be able to perform the task and has already been taught how to complete it.
3. Relatedness – this is where there needs to be an understanding how the learning relates to daily practice and therefore helps to identify the need for the learning.

Box 11.10 outlines some ways in which to motivate learners.

Opportunistic teaching Opportunistic teaching appears self-explanatory, although in this context is being used mainly to discuss teaching in clinical environments (see also Chapter 5). The challenges presented by opportunistic teaching would be that it might not allow for structured planning (Crossland 2021) and therefore setting structured learning objectives might be challenging. Nevertheless, the clinical environment, usually provides unplanned learning opportunities and being ready can help both you as a teacher and the learner. Being ready for unplanned teaching will be helpful, so it will be advisable for you to have a structure for opportunistic teaching. The following steps might be helpful:

Box 11.10 | How to motivate learners

- Be motivated yourself as a teacher
- Be positive, kind and caring
- Set the scene for the teaching – give context and set achievable learning objectives
- Involve learners
- Give constructive and timely feedback
- Give time to learners
- Focus on positives
- Allow time for reflection
- Adapt teaching to learning needs
- Assist learners to take responsibility for their learning

1. Always be aware of when you are being observed or assisting in a clinical procedure. If you have a colleague or learner with you, ask questions such as:
   - Have you participated in such an activity before?
   - Do you know what is happening?
   - What or why do you think the activity is happening?

   By asking these questions, you will be able to help the learner to identify their learning needs.
2. Question the learner further by enquiring why they think the activity is happening and what is their perception or knowledge? This will help to identify the current knowledge baseline and help you to identify what you need to teach.
3. Once you have identified the learning needs, explain the activity and give clear instructions and information. Give a rationale for your explanations as this will then help to reinforce the learning.
4. Once the learner gets more information and knowledge, allow them to participate (within their and your scope of practice) and support them. Appraise and give feedback.
5. Debrief after the learning has happened. This can take the form of you reinforcing the feedback with constructive advice. Explore the feelings of the learner as well and allow for self-reflection.

Teaching clinical skills In addition to role modelling, you will be involved in the teaching of clinical skills to junior colleagues, nursing students and trainee nursing associates. Please remember your scope of practice and be reminded that as a student nurse or trainee nursing associate, you cannot assess the competency of other colleagues.

Learning clinical skills can be seen as multilayered; that is, there is the knowledge aspect (cognitive skills) and the psychomotor aspect

---

Over to you

What is competency?

In simple terms, competence can be described as an ability to perform a task or activity based safely and based on sound standards, knowledge, and evidence. In addition, a competent person must possess the attributes, characteristics, attitude, and skills to be able to meet the requirements of the profession (Fukada 2018). The NMC (2018a) sets the standards for proficiency and competence.

(Mohanna et al. 2011). Burgess et al. (2020) support three main components of teaching clinical skills, which are:

- Knowledge – knowing how and why to perform a skill. This will also involve knowledge and understanding of risks and risk assessments to mitigate these.
- Communication – effective communication needs to be maintained with the patient/client and and ensuring that elements such as informed consent are adhered to.
- Performance – considers the skills required to perform a skill and any preparation which might be required (e.g. setting up an aseptic field prior to performing wound care). It also involves the psychomotor skills required to perform a clinical skill and the post-procedure care that needs to be provided.

Over to you

The application of compression stockings (sometimes called TED – thromboembolus deterrent – stockings) requires appropriate knowledge and the application of appropriate skills. What would you need to consider when teaching a patient or carer with regards to the application of the stockings?

A four-step approach to teaching clinical skills is proposed by Walker and Peyton (1998) (Box 11.11) and expanded further by George and Doto (2001) to a five-step model (Box 11.12). The George and Doto (2001) five-step

Box 11.11 | Four steps approach

1. Demonstration: Instructor demonstrates the skill at normal speed and without additional comments.
2. Deconstruction: Instructor demonstrates the skill by breaking it down into simple steps, while describing each step.
3. Formulation: Instructor demonstrates the skills whilst being 'talked through' the steps by the learner.
4. Performance: Student demonstrates the skill, while describing each step.

Source: Adapted from Walker and Peyton (1998).

> ## Box 11.12 | Five steps to teaching clinical skills
>
> 1. Explain why the skill is needed (eliciting interest)
> 2. Demonstrate
> 3. Demonstrate with commentary
> 4. Learners talk through the procedure
> 5. Learners perform the procedure
>
> *Source:* Adapted from George and Doto (2001).

model adds one extra step – the explaining step, whereby the teacher explains the process by stimulating the interest of the learner (Box 11.12).

Assessment and evaluation

Although as a student nurse/trainee nursing associate you would not formally be assessing colleagues or peers, understanding assessment will help to measure the attainment and success of your teaching. It is important to make the distinction between learner assessment and evaluation and teaching evaluation. We investigate learner assessment briefly and then move on to teaching evaluation.

> ## Write here
>
> Before moving further in this section, spend some time thinking about the differences between learner assessment and evaluation. Jot down some ideas below.

There are subtle differences between assessment and evaluation, although they are sometimes used interchangeably and this can lead to confusion. An assessment can be defined as a systematic process whereby knowledge, skills and understanding can be measured. Assessments are also seen as a means of teaching and learning (Sokhanvar et al. 2021), whereby the process leads to understanding what is already known but also how to apply it in practice and improving current performance. Evaluation, on the other hand, will be an activity of passing judgement based on set standards, guidelines and criteria.

Assessment is an adaptive process; that is, the method of assessment would depend on what was being taught. More recently, concepts such as authentic assessments have become more prominent. Authentic assessments are those where the students are required to use the acquired knowledge applied real-life situations (Wiewiora and Kowalkiewicz 2018).

When you are assessing a learner, you will be measuring to what extent the learning objectives have been achieved hence the importance of setting appropriate SMART objectives at the outset. There are different types of assessment methods, and we cannot explore all of them, but Table 11.3 explores the common methods that you are more likely to use.

TABLE 11.3

Some methods of assessment.

Observation	This will be the most common method of assessment which you will use. Observation is not a simple process, for example, performing a clinical skill correctly does not automatically mean that one is competent. Competence has been described as not directly observable but inferred from successful behaviour (Mohanna et al. 2011). Please remember that there can be two types of observation, either direct observation (when the learner knows they are being observed) and indirect observation.
Peer assessment	Peer assessment would be exactly what you will be doing when you are teaching and assessing a junior colleague or peer. Please remember that peer assessment needs to be structured according to standards and criteria to make it valid and meaningful.
Questioning	Asking questions should not be used as interrogation but needs to be related to the learning objectives and whereby the teacher can assess learning as well as evaluate their own teaching skills.
Reflection and self-assessment	Reflection will form part of your journey from student nurse/trainee nursing associate well into when you are a registered nurse. Reflection in the context of assessment will be where the learner is able to interpret their performance. Through reflection and self-assessment, learners then learn to analyse their own performance, and this can enhance learning but also influence lifelong learning skills (Lidster and Wakefield 2022).

Feedback Once the learner has been assessed either formally or informally, it is essential that timely feedback is given. Feedback has been defined as a process whereby the learner receives insight into their performance (Clynes and Raftery 2008). Feedback is essential as it helps the learner judge their own performance but also more importantly help them set realistic objectives. For feedback to be effective, it is essential that it is timely but also that it is non-judgemental and structured. For feedback to be effective and a learning tool, it is essential that both the learner and teacher form partnerships and become allies in learning (Schartel 2012). Box 11.13 provides some ideas on constructive feedback.

Feedback should not overlap with formal assessment or evaluation of performance; it needs to be formative. Having a structured approach to feedback is advisable and one such structure used is PEARLS (Box 11.14;

Box 11.13 | Characteristics of constructive feedback

- Focus on the content of learning and not the learner
- Be specific and clear,
- Be as simple as possible.
- Unbiased and objective (praise is not feedback).
- Be timed and expected.
- Be regulated with elements that can be rectified.
- Addresses actions and not interpretations.

Box 11.14 | PEARLS

Partnership – there should be a partnership between learner and teacher.

Empathetic – the teacher should show understanding of the learner's needs.

Apology – the teacher should be aware and acknowledge barriers to learning.

Respect – be aware and accept the learner's values and choices.

Legitimation – acknowledge feeling, fears and intentions.

Support – assist the learner on improvement strategies.

Source: Adapted from Milan et al. (2006).

Milan et al. 2006). See also Chapter 10, where feedback and feed forward are also discussed.

Complete this activity now

Spend a few minutes recalling times when you were given feedback. Write down a few of your feelings and emotions when receiving the feedback.

Evaluation Evaluation concerns how to measure the success of the teaching method(s). Evaluation of your own performance is essential for reflection, as you can then judge the success of your performance as a teacher, which then adds to worth and value of methodology (Scriven 1991). Evaluation of teaching will serve three purposes:

1. Measure the effectiveness of teaching methods.
2. Maintain good practice (what works well).
3. Rectify less good practice (what does not work so well).

Evaluation strategies One evaluation strategy measures the skills or knowledge acquisition level of the learner through the assessment process. For example, if the learner can complete taught skills correctly, you can potentially suggest that the teaching methodology worked. However, there would be limitations to using this as a measure of success of your teaching methods. It is possible that the learner already knew the skill or may have learnt it on their own.

Another method of evaluation would be to ask the learner directly whether they felt that the learning was beneficial. However, this can present challenges, as the learner's response could be subject to bias and it is potentially unfair to ask for this type of feedback, as the learner might find it difficult to make known their thoughts in an open and free way.

Indirect evaluation can take several other forms but essentially avoids asking face-to-face questions about the teaching session to the learner. One form of evaluation would be how the learner performs the taught content in their future observable practice. Again, this needs to be used with caution as the methodology might have been correct but the delivery of the teaching content might not have been appropriate.

Another way would be to ask the learner to complete an evaluation form. Not everything can be or needs to be evaluated (Mohanna et al. 2011) and therefore the evaluation form needs to be specific and simple for the learner to complete.

If you are completing a teaching session as an episode of care, likely, you will be observed by a third party, (your practice assessor). In those situations, it would be advisable for you to ensure that you meet your assessor prior to delivering the teaching session and discuss how you plan to deliver the teaching.

Finally, as a teacher, it is also helpful and recommended to maintain your reflective practitioner skills. Being reflective helps the teacher in planning and implementing more effective methods of teaching as well as identifying problems which can then be shared with colleagues (your practice assessor). This can then help identify solutions as well as developing more effective teaching methods (Çimer et al. 2013).

Delegation

As a student teaching peers and other colleagues, there will come a level of delegation which will need to be demonstrated. As you are teaching others, you will therefore be imparting knowledge and skills and as such would have the responsibility to ensure that you are teaching the correct content but also able to ensure correct and safe delegation.

Try this on placement

When you are next on placement, take time to observe how different members of the team are delegated to.

- Who does what in the team and why?
- Who was being delegated to (the delegatee) by the delegator?
- What was the underpinning principle regarding the delegation?
- Who has responsibility for delegating appropriately?

The NMC (2018e) defines delegation 'as the transfer to a competent individual, of the authority to perform a specific task in a specified situation' (Box 11.15).

Box 11.15 | What is delegation?

Delegation of an activity may be from:

- one registered professional to another
- a registered professional to an unregulated member of staff
- a registered or unregistered person to a carer or family member.

As a student nurse/trainee nursing associate you will not yet be a registered professional, but you will still have to abide by the NMC Code.

Source: Adapted from NMC (2018e).

Delegation usually involves at least two individuals: the delegator, and the delegatee (Barrow and Sharma 2021). Three other aspects can be identified namely:

1. Responsibility – as someone accepting to complete a delegated task, you are responsible for your actions.
2. Authority – one needs to be in a position of authority to be able to delegate. For example, in your episode of care, you would have discussed the teaching episode with your practice assessor and should have been deemed as competent in delivering the session.
3. Accountability – you as a teacher are then accountable for any delegated task.

The five rights of delegation (American Nurses Association, 2019) are identified in Box 11.16 below. The NMC Code (NMC 2018e) sets out the responsibilities of people on the register when they accept a delegated task (Box 11.17).

Box 11.16 | Five rights of delegation

- Right task
- Right circumstance
- Right person
- Right directions and communication
- Right supervision and evaluation

Source: Adapted from National Council of State Boards of Nursing and American Nurses Association (2019).

Box 11.17 | Responsibilities in delegation

- Make sure that patient and public safety is not affected. You work within the limits of your competence, exercising your professional 'duty of candour' and raising concerns immediately whenever you come across situations that put patients or public safety at risk
- Make a timely referral to another practitioner when any action, care or treatment is required.
- Ask for help from a suitably qualified and experienced health and care professional to carry out any action or procedure that is beyond the limits of your competence.
- Complete the necessary training before carrying out a new role.

Source: Adapted from NMC (2018e).

Summary

This chapter has introduced many concepts of pedagogy and andragogy and has hopefully warmed up your appetite to learn more about teaching. Nursing, as your chosen profession, will be a lifelong learning process and you will be taught and will be teaching others throughout your nursing career and possibly beyond.

A key focus of this chapter has been on writing learning objectives. Planning and structuring teaching are also key elements for both teaching and learning to become effective. There is no perfect teaching methodology, just as there is no perfect learning theory, and the key is to be adaptable and willing to change methodologies when needed.

Teachers should use a reflective process and acknowledge that the individual is always learning and making positive changes and learning remains lifelong.

References

Abela, J. (2009). Adult learning theories and medical education: a review. *Malta Medical Journal* 21: 11–18.

Baldwin, A., Mills, J., Birks, M., and Budden, L. (2014). Role modeling in undergraduate nursing education: an integrative literature review. *Nurse Education Today* 34 (6): e18–e26.

Bandura, A. (1977). Self-efficacy: toward a unifying theory of behavioral change. *Psychological Review* 84 (2): 191–215.

Barrow, J.M. and Sharma, S. (2021). *Five Rights of Nursing Delegation*. Treasure Island (FL): StatPearls Publishing. https://www.ncbi.nlm.nih.gov/books/NBK519519 (accessed:10 August 2022).

Bezanilla, M.J., Fernández-Nogueira, D., Poblete, M., and Galindo-Domínguez, H. (2019). Methodologies for teaching-learning critical thinking in higher education: the teacher's view. *Thinking Skills and Creativity* 33: 1–10.

Biggs, J.B. and Collis, K.F. (1982). *Evaluating the Quality of Learning: The SOLO Taxonomy (Structure of the Observed Learning Outcome)*. New York, NY: Academic Press.

Bloom, B.S. (1956). *Taxonomy of Educational Objectives, Handbook: The Cognitive Domain*. New York, NY: David McKay.

Bond, M. and Holland, S. (2011). *Skills of Clinical Supervision for Nurses: A Practical Guide for Supervisees, Clinical Supervisors, and Managers*. London: McGraw-Hill Education.

Burgess, A., van Diggele, C., Roberts, C. et al. (2020). Tips for teaching procedural skills. *BMC Medical Education* 20 (Suppl 2): 458. https://doi.org/10.1186/s12909-020-02284-1.

Bye, D., Pushkar, D., and Conway, M. (2007). Motivation, interest, and positive affect in traditional and non-traditional undergraduate students. *Adult Education Quarterly* 57: 141–158.

Çimer, A., Çimer, S.O., Sezen, G., and Vekli, S. (2013). How does reflection help teachers to become effective teachers? *International Journal of Educational Research* 1 (4): 133–149.

Clynes, M.P. and Raftery, S.E.C. (2008). Feedback: an essential element of student learning in clinical practice. *Nurse Education in Practice* 8: 405–411.

Crossland, C. (2021). Teaching in the clinical environment. *Update in Anaesthesia* 36: 13–17.

Dewey, J. (1984). *Individualism Old and New*. New York, NY: Prometheus Books.

Education Scotland (2005) *Let's talk about Pedagogy*: Towards a shared understanding for early years education in Scotland. Edinburgh: Learning and Teaching Scotland. https://education.gov.scot/media/13khv2ys/talkpedagogy.pdf (accessed 31 July 2022).

Fink, L.D. (2003). *Creating Significant Learning Experiences: An Integrated Approach to Designing College Courses*. San Francisco, CA: Jossey-Bass.

Fukada, M. (2018). Nursing competency: definition, structure and development. *Yonago Acta Medica* 61 (1): 1–7.

Gardner, H.E. (2000). *Intelligence Reframed: Multiple Intelligences for the 21st Century*. London: Hachette.

George, G.H. and Doto, F.X. (2001). A simple five-step method for teaching clinical skills. *Family Medicine* 33 (8): 577–578.

International Bureau of Education (2022) *Most influential theories of learning*. General Education System Quality Analysis/Diagnosis Framework. Geneva: UNESCO. http://www.ibe.unesco.org/en/geqaf/annexes/technical-notes/most-influential-theories-learning (accessed 29 July 2022).

Jacobsen, T.-I., Sandsleth, M.G., and Gonzalez, M.T. (2022). Student nurses' experiences participating in a peer mentoring program in clinical placement studies: a metasynthesis. *Nurse Education in Practice* 61: 1–10.

Knowles, M.S. (1980). *The Modern Practice of Adult Education: From Pedagogy to Andragogy*. York, NY: Cambridge.

Landøy, A., Popa, D., and Repanovici, A. (2019). *Teaching Learning Methods*. Cham: Springer Open.

Lidster, J. and Wakefield, S. (2022). *Student Practice Supervision and Assessment*, 2e. London: Sage.

Maynard, E., Helga Stittrich-Lyons, H., and Emery, C. (2016). "You share a coffee, you share cases": the professional experiences of safeguarding in universal praxis. In: *Rethinking Social Issues in Education for the 21st Century: UK Perspectives on International Concerns*, 2e (ed. W. Sims-Schouten and S. Horton), 2–25. Newcastle upon Tyne: Cambridge Scholars.

Milan, F.B., Parish, S.J., and Reichgott, M.J. (2006). A model for educational feedback based on clinical communication skills strategies: beyond the feedback sandwich. *Teaching and Learning in Medicine* 18: 42–47.

Mohanna, K., Cottrell, E., Wall, D., and Chambers, D. (2011). *Teaching Made Easy*, 3e. Oxford: Radcliffe.

Murphy, F. (2006). Motivation in nurse education practice: a case study approach. *British Journal of Nursing* 15 (20): 1132–1135.

Murray, C.J. and Main, A. (2005). Role modelling as a teaching method for student mentors. *Nursing Times* 101 (26): 30–33.

National Council of State Boards of Nursing, American Nurses Association (2019). *National Guidelines for Nursing Delegation*. Chicago, IL: NCSBS and ANA. https://www.ncsbn.org/nursing-regulation/practice/delegation.page (accessed 10 August 2022).

Noor, N.M., Harunb, J., and Arisa, B. (2012). Andragogy and pedagogy learning model preference among undergraduate students. *Procedia – Social and Behavioral Sciences* 56 (8): 673–678.

Nursing and Midwifery Council (2018a). *Future Nurse: Standards of Proficiency for Registered Nurses*. London: NMC.

Nursing and Midwifery Council (2018b). *Part 1: Standards Framework for Nursing and Midwifery Education*. London: NMC.

Nursing and Midwifery Council (2018c). *The Code: Professional Standards of Practice and Behaviour for Nurses, Midwives and Nursing Associates*. London: NMC.

Nursing and Midwifery Council (2018d). *Part 3: Standards for Pre-Registration*. London: NMC.

Nursing and Midwifery Council (2018e). *Delegation and accountability: Supplementary information to the NMC code*. London: NMC. www.nmc.org.uk/globalassets/sitedocuments/nmc-publications/delegation-and-accountability-supplementary-information-to-the-nmc-code.pdf (accessed 10 August 2022).

Nursing and Midwifery Council (2022). *Our role in education*. www.nmc.org.uk/education/our-role-in-education (accessed 28 July 2022).

Pan London Practice Learning Group (2021). *Pan London e-PAD: project update*. PLPLG Newsletter (12). https://plplg.uk/wp-content/uploads/2021/07/PLPLG_Newsletter_A4_Issue-12_v5.pdf

Pew, S. (2007). Andragogy and pedagogy as foundational theory for student motivation in higher education. *Student Motivation* 2: 14–25.

Prozescky, D.R. (2000). Teaching and learning. *Community Eye Health* 13 (34): 30–31.

Rachal, J.R. (2002). Andragogy's detectives: a critique of the present and proposal for the future. *Adult Education Quarterly* 52 (3): 210–227.

Rajagopalan, I. (2019). Concept of teaching. *International Journal of Education* 7 (2): 5–8.

Rogers, C. (1951). *Client-centered Therapy: Its current practice, implications and theory.* London: Constable.

Ryan, R.M. and Deci, E.L. (2000). Intrinsic and extrinsic motivations: classic definitions and new directions. *Contemporary Educational Psychology* 25 (1): 54–67.

Saab, M.M., Kilty, C., Meehan, E. et al. (2021). Peer group clinical supervision: qualitative perspectives from nurse supervisees, managers, and supervisors. *Collegian* 4: 359–368.

Schartel, S.A. (2012). Giving feedback: an integral part of education. *Best Practice and Research Clinical Anaesthesiology* 26: 77–87.

Scriven, S. (1991). *Evaluation Thesaurus*, 4e. Newbury Park: Sage.

Sokhanvar, Z., Salehi, K., and Sokhanvar, F. (2021). Advantages of authentic assessment for improving the learning experience and employability skills of higher education students: a systematic literature review. *Studies in Educational Evaluation* 70: 1–10.

Tuma, F. and Nassar, A.K. (2021). Applying Bloom's taxonomy in clinical surgery: practical examples. *Annals of Medicine and Surgery* 69: 1–3.

University and College Union (2009). *UCU's vision of adult learning.* London: UCU. https://www.ucu.org.uk/adultlearning_UCUvision (accessed 28 July 2022).

Walker, M. and Peyton, J.W.R. (1998). *Teaching in Theatre. Teaching and Learning in Medical Practice.* Rickmansworth: Manticore Europe.

Wiewiora, A. and Kowalkiewicz, A. (2018). The role of authentic assessment in developing authentic leadership identity and competencies. *Assessment and Evaluation in Higher Education* 43: 415–430.

Wiggins, G. and McTighe, J. (2005). *Understanding by Design*, 2e. Alexandria, VA: Association for Supervision and Curriculum Development.

CHAPTER 12

Lifelong learning

Catherine Jones and Kim Lewin

AIM

This chapter provides the reader with an understanding of lifelong learning in a professional context and review the requirements of the Nursing and Midwifery Council (NMC) for revalidation.

LEARNING OUTCOMES

1. Describe the importance of lifelong learning to professional practice.
2. Understand the revalidation requirements for professional registration with the NMC:
   - Practice hours
   - Continuing professional development (CPD)
   - Practice-related feedback
   - Written reflective accounts
   - Reflective discussion
   - Health and character
   - Professional indemnity insurance
   - Confirmation.
3. Demonstrate awareness of processes and documentation associated with revalidation.

Succeeding on your Nursing Placement: Supervision, Learning and Assessment for Nursing Students, First Edition. Edited by Ian Peate.
© 2024 John Wiley & Sons Ltd. Published 2024 by John Wiley & Sons Ltd.

Introduction

Other chapters in this book have considered how learners learn, opportunities for learning in practice and how feedback and feedforward can enhance the care that our service users experience. We hope that you are already starting to think about the ways in which you can make the most of opportunities in clinical placement to develop your own professional practice. In this chapter, the emphasis shifts to what happens after you register and ways to embed the learning attributes that you have developed as a student to nourish and sustain your practice after registration. The concept of lifelong learning is outlined and discussed with reference to the professional context. NMC revalidation requirements are outlined (See Figure 12.1) and discussed in detail. Relevant documentation and processes will be highlighted throughout this discussion.

Lifelong learning

Nurses and other healthcare professionals work in complex clinical environments that are constantly evolving. As future clinicians, we should agree that the development of up-to-date knowledge and skills and evidence-based working practices can only be of benefit to patient care. With that in mind, lifelong learning can be defined as: 'formal and informal learning opportunities that allow you to continuously develop and improve the knowledge and skills you need for employment and personal fulfilment' (Interprofessional CPD and Lifelong Learning UK Working Group 2019).

Lifelong learning has been in the consciousness of the nursing profession for as long as there have been professional nurses. A quote attributed to Florence Nightingale encapsulates this view: 'Let us never consider ourselves finished nurses . . . We must be learning all of our lives'.

The NMC supports and advocates lifelong learning for all nurses and midwives and requires evidence of CPD for the mandatory renewal of professional registration. However, while now enshrined in the standards for professional revalidation and considered a fundamental part of nursing practice, lifelong learning has not always been such a formalised requirement for nurses. As such, it is useful to understand the context for the mandating of standards for lifelong learning, both within nursing education and within the wider health and social care arena.

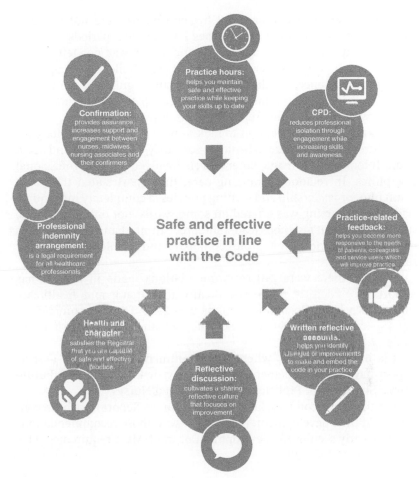

FIGURE 12.1 Safe and effective practice. *Source:* NMC (2019) How to revalidate with the NMC. Available from: https://www.nmc.org.uk/globalassets/sitedocuments/revalidation/how-to-revalidate-booklet.pdf (accessed 3 June 2022).

The Francis Report

In 2013, the findings of a public inquiry into Mid Staffordshire NHS Foundation Trust were published. The inquiry, which became known as the Francis Report, was chaired by Robert Francis QC, and investigated the care provided to patients at the trust's hospital site, following concerns raised regarding the trust's mortality rates compared with other similar trusts. The report makes for sobering reading, describing incidents where patients' personal hygiene needs were not met and patients were left in soiled bed clothes for extended periods, patients were not supported to eat and drink and water was not left within patients reach. Patients were not assisted with toileting, in spite of requesting assistance, standards for privacy and dignity were not maintained, even in death and staff appeared to treat patients and those close to them with 'callous indifference' (Francis 2013).

The Francis Report went on to look at why it had taken so long for the failures in patient care to be taken seriously, investigated and acted upon. It looked at all management levels involved and all professional disciplines. In relation to nursing care, the report stated that, as a result of poor leadership and staffing policies, a completely inadequate standard of nursing was offered on some wards: not only inadequate staffing levels but also poor leadership, recruitment and training. This in turn led to declining professionalism and a tolerance of poor standards.

In total, there were 290 recommendations made in the Francis Report, of which 29 relate specifically to nursing and healthcare support workers (Recommendations 185–213). Those recommendations specifically related to nurses' education and learning are listed in Table 12.1.

It is important to see where the recommendations of the Francis Report have been implemented. If you revisit Chapter 2 and Future Nurse: Standards of Proficiency for Registered Nurses (NMC, 2018a), it is clear that the recommendations of the Francis Report have been considered in their development. In the same way, those recommendations can be clearly seen in the development of the NMC's requirements for revalidation (NMC 2019).

Go online

Take some time to read the full Francis Report: https://www.gov.uk/government/publications/report-of-the-mid-staffordshire-nhs-foundation-trust-public-inquiry

Jot down some notes on what this report means for you as an individual and as a future registered professional.

Lifelong learning is not a concept that is isolated to the nursing profession alone. The Interprofessional CPD and Lifelong Learning UK Working Group, comprising representatives across health and social care

TABLE 12.1

Recommendations from the Francis Report (nursing training and learning).

No.	Theme	Recommendation	Chapter
185	Focus on culture of caring	There should be an increased focus in nurse training, education and professional development on the practical requirements of delivering compassionate care in addition to the theory. A system which ensures the delivery of proper standards of nursing requires: • Selection of recruits to the profession who evidence the: ◦ Possession of the appropriate values, attitudes and behaviours; ◦ Ability and motivation to enable them to put the welfare of others above their own interests; ◦ Drive to maintain, develop and improve their own standards and abilities; ◦ Intellectual achievements to enable them to acquire through training the necessary technical skills; • Training and experience in delivery of compassionate care; • Leadership which constantly reinforces values and standards of compassionate care; • Involvement in, and responsibility for, the planning and delivery of compassionate care; • Constant support and incentivisation which values nurses and the work they do through: Recognition of achievement; Regular, comprehensive feedback on performance and concerns; Encouraging them to report concerns and to give priority to patient well-being.	23

(Continued)

TABLE 12.1

(Continued)

No.	Theme	Recommendation	Chapter
186	Practical hands-on training and experience	Nursing training should be reviewed so that sufficient practical elements are incorporated to ensure that a consistent standard is achieved by all trainees throughout the country. This requires national standards.	23
189	Consistent training	The Nursing and Midwifery Council and other professional and academic bodies should work towards a common qualification assessment/examination.	23
190	National standards	There should be national training standards for qualification as a registered nurse to ensure that newly qualified nurses are competent to deliver a consistent standard to the fundamental aspects of compassionate care.	23
193	Standards for appraisal and support	Without introducing a revalidation scheme immediately, the Nursing and Midwifery Council should introduce common minimum standards for appraisal and support with which responsible others would be obliged to comply. They could be required to report to the Nursing and Midwifery Council on their performance on a regular basis.	23
194		As part of a mandatory annual performance appraisal, each Nurse, regardless of workplace setting, should be required to demonstrate in their annual learning portfolio an up-to-date knowledge of nursing practice and its implementation. Alongside developmental requirements, this should contain documented evidence of recognised training undertaken, including wider relevant learning. It should also demonstrate commitment, compassion and caring for patients, evidenced by feedback from patients and families on the care provided by the nurse. This portfolio and each annual appraisal should be made available to the Nursing and Midwifery Council, if requested, as part of a nurse's revalidation process.	23

> **TABLE 12.1**
>
> **(Continued)**

No.	Theme	Recommendation	Chapter
		At the end of each annual assessment, the appraisal and portfolio should be signed by the nurse as being an accurate and true reflection and be countersigned by their appraising manager as being such.	
197		Training and continuing professional development for nurses should include leadership training at every level from student to director. A resource for nurse leadership training should be made available for all NHS healthcare provider organisations that should be required under commissioning arrangements by those buying healthcare services to arrange such training for appropriate staff.	23

Source: Francis (2013)/TSO a Williams Lea company/public domain (OGL).

(including the Royal College of Nursing and the Royal College of Midwives) developed a set of principles in 2019 that focus on the standards for lifelong learning and recognise the importance of CPD for both the accomplishment of professional duties and individuals' own sense of fulfilment.

According to the Interprofessional CPD and Lifelong Learning UK Working Group (2019), it is recognised that a unified approach to developing an appropriately resourced and clinically effective workforce will raise the quality of care provided and have the added benefits of lowering clinical risk and improving clinical outcomes. The five principles of CPD and lifelong learning are that they should:

1. Be each person's responsibility and be made possible and supported by your employer.
2. Benefit the service users.
3. Improve the quality of service delivery.
4. Be balanced and relevant to each person's area of practice or employment.
5. Be recorded and show the effect on each person's area of practice.

Over to you

Before you read on, take a moment to brainstorm what you think the benefits of CPD and lifelong learning might be for you, your service users, and the organisations within which you are going to work.

Benefit to me	Benefit to service users	Benefit to the organisation

Each of the five principles is broken down into three roles: those of you, the individual, your employer and the wider system. This helps to demonstrate the importance of functioning employers and systems to the development of the individual. This can be seen in principle 1, which describes the responsibilities of these roles in relation to CPD and lifelong learning (Table 12.2).

While your employer and the wider system should provide opportunities, this approach places the responsibility back on the individual (you!) to plan, prioritise and engage with and reflect on CPD activities to inform your own lifelong learning. If you refer to the beginning of the chapter and consider the definition of lifelong learning, it becomes clear that you are best placed to know what it is you need to learn to develop yourself. CPD includes both planned formalised activities, such as training courses and conference or webinar attendance, as well as informal, spontaneous opportunities for learning such as debrief on clinical situations in practice.

Try this on placement

When you are next out on placement, take the opportunity to see what formal learning opportunities are available to the staff and what less structured/informal opportunities there are for learning and CPD. Are there activities you are undertaking on which you can reflect to showcase your own personal and professional learning?

TABLE 12.2

The three roles associated with lifelong learning and continuing professional development (principle 1).

Principle 1: Be each person's responsibility and be made possible and supported by your employer

You	• You are responsible for regularly planning, prioritising, carrying out, applying and reflecting on CPD and lifelong learning. • You appreciate and recognise that valuable learning can happen in both planned and unplanned situations. • You are responsible for identifying and demonstrating the benefits of learning to influence and gain support from your employer (if this applies).
Your employer	• Has a responsibility to make sure that you are safe, up to date with current practices and can meet the needs of service users, in line with your professional standards. • Provides fair access to time, study leave and funding to allow you to: Plan learning Carry out learning, and Think about the outcomes of learning. • Encourages and supports access to learning that is separate to statutory and compulsory training, for the benefit of service users. Provides and supports access to resources (for example, technology) when they are needed.
The wider system	Is responsible for creating and promoting opportunities for integrated learning across teams.

Source: Interprofessional CPD and Lifelong Learning UK Working Group (2019).

Now you have had an opportunity to consider the responsibility you have for your own learning, it is important to link that learning back to our patients (Table 12.3).

While principle 1 places the individual front and centre at identifying their own learning needs, it is vital that any proposed learning activity should be relevant to the care of the patient group you are involved with supporting. For example, you might have an interest in learning more about child immunisation, but this would be of limited relevance if you are providing care to adult patients in an intensive care setting. Considering the relevance of the training it is also necessary to gain approval for the requisite funding and study leave to undertake these activities.

TABLE 12.3

The three roles associated with lifelong learning and continuing professional development (principle 2).

Principle 2: Benefit the service users

You	• Your learning should develop new knowledge and skills, add to your existing skills, and provide opportunities to initiate and reinforce best practice. • Your learning should be relevant to the needs of your service users or your employer (or both) and used in your area of practice.
Your employer	• Is responsible for identifying the needs of service users to guide how relevant your learning is.
The wider system	• Is responsible for supporting and promoting quality CPD and lifelong learning that benefits service users.

Source: Interprofessional CPD and Lifelong Learning UK Working Group (2019).

Over to you

Think back to what you identified in the previous 'Try this on placement' exercise. Consider how you might be able to provide a rationale for why it is relevant to your patient care to obtaining a place on that training activity. This is good practice for when you become a registrant, as you are more likely to have your requests for CPD approved if you are able to provide a clear rationale for them.

Let us move on to consider principle 3 (Table 12.4) and the quality of the services we provide to our patients and service users. As you can see from Table 12.4, principle 3 takes the points from principle 2 and expands on them. Considering our role as thoughtful clinical practitioners, it is also vital to take into consideration how our CPD is rooted in evidence-based practice, so it is important to have researched any planned learning activities, have a clear idea of whether they are evidence based and how proposed activities will benefit the service in which you are working and improve the quality of care that is being provided.

> **TABLE 12.4**
>
> ## The three roles associated with lifelong learning and continuing professional development (principle 3).
>
> **Principle 3: Improve the quality of service delivery**
>
> | | |
> |---|---|
> | You | • You explore and use ways to show how your learning has improved the quality of your practice.
• Your learning and the outcomes of your learning improve the quality of your service delivery and reduce risk.
• You identify opportunities to learn from and share learning with others. |
> | Your employer | • Encourages a culture of learning from experiences with positive outcomes, as well as from situations that did not go well.
• Supports learning opportunities between individuals, teams and networks, across services and organisations.
• Supports learning activity with time, staffing and resources to improve the quality of their service. |
> | The wider system | • Provides resources for quality learning through management, workforce and service delivery plans.
• Evaluates the effect of an appropriately qualified workforce on the quality of services.
• Has systems in place to assess the quality of CPD and lifelong learning activity |
>
> *Source:* Interprofessional CPD and Lifelong Learning UK Working Group (2019).

Complete this activity now

Conduct a search of CPD courses which you think may be relevant to your practice. This could be online or using a printed prospectus. Are you able to see any reference to literature which suggests that the educational activity is evidence based? Does this impact on whether you may want to undertake the training/educational activity?

While health and social care has historically followed discipline specific roles and professional development, there is now a consensus that professionals should also have a broader understanding of the wider health and social care landscape, as there is a lot that can be improved with shared knowledge and understanding. Principle 4 (Table 12.5) makes this explicit.

Across the four areas identified in principle 4 (health and social care, learning and education, leadership and evidence, research and development; Table 12.5), it should now be apparent that all these areas are relevant to the care of our patients, whatever discipline or field of health and social care we are working in. For example, if

---

TABLE 12.5

The three roles associated with lifelong learning and CPD (principle 4).

Principle 4: Be balanced and relevant to each person's area of practice or employment

You	• Your learning should include activities across the following four areas: Health and social care Learning and education Leadership Evidence, research and development. • You take part in a range of learning activities, both formal and informal, as well as active and reflective (where you think about what you have learned). • You take part in learning that is relevant to, challenges and develops your current or intended area of practice. • Your learning meets relevant organisational, professional or regulatory standards.
Your employer	• Recognises and supports learning across the following four areas: Health and social care Learning and education Leadership Evidence, research and development. • Provides opportunities for a range of learning, including employees learning with and from each other. • Responds to your learning needs within a constantly changing, challenging and complex environment.
The wider system	• Promotes the value of a range of learning activities.Recognises and reinforces that the most important parts of learning are the outcomes.

Source: Interprofessional CPD and Lifelong Learning UK Working Group (2019).

working as a community staff nurse, you may work on a daily basis with people who face challenges around their *social care* needs, which has an impact on whether they are able to engage with their own health needs and self-management. It may be very useful to you, both for your own development and to provide quality evidence-based care, to access training around social care assessment and provision within your local area.

In the same way, a staff nurse on a busy surgical ward may work regularly with student nurses, trainee nursing associates and health care assistants and may identify a learning need for themselves that further formal education and training in learning and education would enable them to better support the students in practice and potentially increase the likelihood of recruitment from that student group. While not a clinical skill, this has potential benefits for the individual, the students on the ward and the patients being looked after.

Over to you

Take a few minutes to look at these four areas. Based on your experience so far, jot down any types of learning from within these areas you feel might be beneficial to you in the future:

Health and social care
Learning and education
Leadership
Evidence, research and development

TABLE **12.6**

The three roles associated with lifelong learning and CPD (principle 5).

Principle 5: Be recorded and show the effect on each person's area of practice	
You	• You are responsible for keeping a record of your learning that demonstrates: • what you learnthow it adds to or develops your area of practice, and • the effect on service users or service delivery. • You are responsible for accessing, promoting and using the resources available to you to support your CPD and lifelong learning. • You are responsible for making sure you respect service users' confidentiality.
Your employer	• Provides time, resources and opportunities to allow you to record and think about the outcomes of learning. • Provides the opportunity to share the outcomes of learning across organisations. • Has systems in place to monitor and audit fair access to CPD and lifelong learning activity.
The wider system	• Raises awareness of existing and new resources to support recording and thinking about the outcome of learning.

Source: Interprofessional CPD and Lifelong Learning UK Working Group (2019).

In professional life, we develop skills in documenting our activities with patients as part of our professional responsibilities. Principle 5 (Table 12.6) advocates the same approach to our learning end development.

When recording the evidence of your learning, it is important to follow the guidance of the regulator. For registered nurses and nursing associates, that is the NMC. We go on to discuss the requirements for professional revalidation in the next section.

Revalidation

As previously discussed, the NMC is the independent body responsible for the professional regulation of nurses, midwives, and nursing associates in England. The NMC requires all registrants (nurses, midwives, and nursing associates) to renew their professional registration every three years. Revalidation is the process through which this can be achieved and enables registrants to maintain their registration with the NMC. Registrants are required to 'revalidate' every three years and the NMC will write to registrants to advise when this is due. Registrants must maintain a record that aligns to the revalidation requirements over the entire three-year period to demonstrate their ongoing engagement with Lifelong learning.

Green flag

Revalidation is not an assessment of fitness to practise. There are different processes available to raise concerns about a registrant's fitness to practise.

The revalidation processes require registrants to demonstrate that they are still able to practise safely and provide evidence of their continued development and lifelong learning throughout their career (NMC 2019)

A supervisor's notes

When I first heard about the introduction of revalidation in 2017, I was nervous, and a bit concerned about all the extra work that it would mean. I work full time and have three kids so I couldn't really see where it would fit in. The hospital that I work in did some training sessions to explain it all so things became clearer after that. I realised that it was just formalising things that I already like to do to keep myself up to date. I like the freedom that it gives me to use things that are meaningful to me. For example, I am an infection control link nurse, so I used our hand hygiene audit as part of my practice related feedback. I then used this feedback as the basis for one of my five reflections and was able to identify some action points to develop my own practice as an infection control link nurse and my team's practice in terms of hand hygiene. I also really like that the reflective accounts ask you to reflect with the Code in mind. Before revalidation, we didn't talk about the Code very much unless someone had done something wrong. Now, it is part of our everyday language and considerations, and I really like that. As far as fitting it all in, I find the trick is to be organised and gather your materials over the whole three years.

As registered nurses or nursing associates, we are subject to the professional standards detailed in the Code (NMC 2018b). Revalidation aims to increase awareness of the Code and the professional standards that we can expect practitioners on the professional register to uphold. Registrants should reflect on the role of the Code in their everyday practice and what it means to them. It is hoped that this emphasis on reflection should encourage a professional culture that shares good practice and continuous improvement. Revalidation helps registrants to remain up to date and maintain their professional practice at a standard which will enable them to respond to the changes in healthcare and the needs of their service users. If all the above are achieved, it is hoped that revalidation should lead to consistent and safe practice that is aligned to the professional Code. This should in turn serve to protect the public from unnecessary harm and/or concern. The NMC (2019) requires registrants to show evidence of the following when revalidating:

- practice hours
- CPD
- practice-related feedback
- written reflective accounts
- reflective discussion
- health and character
- professional indemnity insurance
- confirmation.

Practice hours

The practice hours requirement gives registrants the opportunity to record their practice hours in whatever settings they are working in and enables them to demonstrate that they are maintaining safe practices and an up-to-date skills profile over the three-year revalidation period (NMC 2019; Table 12.7).

Practice hours should be carefully documented to ensure an accurate record that includes the following elements:

- dates of practice
- number of hours
- name, address, and postcode of the organisation(s)
- scope of practice, work setting, and brief description of work undertaken
- evidence of practice hours (NMC 2019).

TABLE 12.7

Practice hours.

Registration	Minimum total practice hours required
Nurse	450
Midwife	450
Nursing associate	450
Nurse and specialist community public health nurse	450
Midwife and specialist community public health nurse	450
Nurse and midwife	900 450 (for nursing) 450 (for midwifery)
Nursing associate and nurse	900 450 (for nursing associate) 450 (for nursing)

Source: Adapted from NMC (2019).

It is not necessary to document individual practice hours (e.g. individual shifts) but practice hours should be reported using standard working days, hours per week, to clearly document a minimum of 450 hours (for a registered nurse, midwife or nursing associate).

Go online

The NMC has provided a useful template that is recommended to help registrants log their practice hours. Practice Hours Log Template: www. nmc.org.uk/revalidation/resources/forms-and-templates

It should be emphasised that practice hours completed prior to registering with the NMC do not count towards your practice hours (NMC 2019). Practice hours can only be logged when you work in a role that depends on your expertise and skills as a nurse, midwife or nursing associate (NMC 2019). Hours completed in healthcare assistant, nursing or midwifery assistant or support worker role cannot be counted towards your practice hours as a registered nurse, midwife or nursing associate (NMC 2019).

If registrants are unable to meet the requirements for practice hours because they have not worked in a role that relied on expertise and skills as nurse, midwife or nursing associate or do not have enough hours working in such a position, there are two options:

1. Complete an NMC approved Return to Practice programme
2. Cancel NMC registration. This will lapse the professional registration and will prevent the nurse, midwife or nursing associate from practising (NMC 2019).

If you are not practising in a role that requires your expertise and skills as a nurse, midwife or nursing associate at the point of revalidation but have achieved the required number of hours, details of the most recent practice (including scope of practice and work setting) can be submitted to meet this element of revalidation (NMC 2019).

Try this on placement

When you are in clinical placement, try logging your hours using the NMC template. Think about what kind of work setting you are in: do the labels given on the template describe your placement area? Think about the scope of practice you are involved with on this placement. Ask your practice assessor or supervisor how they describe their work setting and scope of practice for revalidation and see if it matches your own.

Continuous professional development

All practitioners should learn through their everyday activities at work. CPD relates to learning that occurs in addition to those everyday activities. Patients and service users expect registrants to care for them using knowledge and skills that are current and based on recent evidence. CPD and lifelong learning help registrants to achieve these skills (NMC 2019). This approach also enables practitioners to acquire new skills and knowledge in response to changes in healthcare provision, new and evolving evidence and the needs of service users (NMC 2019; Table 12.8).

TABLE **12.8**

Continuous professional development.

Requirement	Supporting evidence
35 hours of continuing professional development (of which 20 must be participatory)	Maintain accurate and verifiable records of your CPD activities, including: • the CPD method (examples of 'CPD method' are self-learning, online learning, course) • a brief description of the topic and how it relates to your scope of practice • dates the CPD activity was undertaken • the number of hours and participatory hours • identification of the part of the Code most relevant to the CPD, and • you should record evidence of the CPD activity.

Source: Adapted from NMC (2019).

While the NMC mandates a minimum of 35 hours of CPD, there is no upper limit on the number of hours that can be recorded. It is important to keep records of the CPD activities undertaken as the evidence required can be difficult to put together weeks, months or years after it has taken place, making it more difficult to revalidate.

Go online

The NMC has provided a useful template that is recommended to help registrants log their continuing professional development. CPD Log Template: www.nmc.org.uk/revalidation/resources/forms-and-templates

This requirement stipulates that 20 of the mandated 35 hours should be in participatory learning. Participatory learning refers to activities where registrants personally interact with other learners in the hope of reducing professional isolation and sustaining networks that share good practice (NMC 2019). This interaction does not always need to take place in a physical space, it can also occur in online forums such as discussion groups or interactive webinars.

Go online

For an example of participatory learning, see the Twitter feed #WeNurses: https://twitter.com/WeNurses

Participatory learning is an effective way to explore new ideas and practices together with other professionals and think about how developments can be implemented into an individual's professional practice. We can learn a great deal from our colleagues working in other geographical locations in the UK and internationally or in other clinical settings.

Although there is no specific type of CPD mandated by the NMC, it is important that any learning activity should have clear links to the registrant's current scope of practice (NMC 2019). Mandatory training is an essential activity for most registrants to meet statutory and corporate obligations. Mandatory training should only be logged as CPD if it has direct relevance to the individual's current scope of practice, e.g. infection prevention and control training for registrants involved with direct clinical care (NMC 2019). There are many opportunities available to registrants to develop knowledge and skills relevant to their scope of practice. Sometimes it is necessary to be creative and versatile in the approach that is taken to developing and maintaining the knowledge and skills to inform their practice. It is important that CPD has meaning and can be applied in the registrants' everyday activities at work (NMC 2019).

The NMC (2021a) has provided some examples of CPD and how to provide evidence of the activity to get you started (Table 12.9). It is acknowledged that it is not always easy to keep abreast of all that is happening in health and social care as things move quickly and the landscape is constantly changing. Subscribing to updates is a way of helping to keep you updated.

Go online

The following websites are particularly useful professional resources and have a subscription facility:

- NMC: you can sign up to receive the nurses and nursing associate's newsletter at: www.nmc.org.uk/news/email-newsletters

- National Institute for Health and Care Excellence: you can subscribe to get alerts and updates regarding publications and new guidance: www.nice.org.uk/news/nice-newsletters-and-alerts
- Department of Health and Social Care: you can subscribe to a range of updates on different areas depending on your areas of clinical interest at: https://dhsc-mail.co.uk/form/Sx1iaZDJ/lf1PJ8tkL/dhsc-email-sign-up
- King's Fund: you can subscribe to a range of updates on new recommendations and studies which may influence health and social care policy at: www.kingsfund.org.uk/emails?utm_source=button

TABLE **12.9**

Examples of continuing professional development activity.

CPD activity	Supporting evidence	Individual/ participatory
Structured learning (direct or distance learning style)	Certificate of completion, notes, learning outcomes	Individual/participatory
Accredited college or university level education or training	Certificate of completion, notes, learning outcomes	Individual/participatory
Learning events such as workshops, conferences	Certificate of attendance	Participatory
Reading and reviewing publications	Copies of publications read, review notes including practice related outcomes	Individual
Coaching and mentoring in a specific skill (role in either delivery or being a recipient)	Evidence of coaching and mentoring undertaken including letters, notes, observations and practice related outcomes	Participatory
Group or practice meetings outside of everyday practice (e.g. to discuss a specific event or new way of working)	Evidence of participation and role including signed letters, notes, observations and outcomes	Participatory

Source: Adapted from NMC (2021a).

When considering what type of CPD will be most useful to help you to develop your practice, the NMC (2019) encourages registrants to look at the most recent standards of proficiency. CPD activities should be undertaken that help registrants to develop skills to meet the requirements of the new proficiencies that have relevance to the practitioners' scope of practice (NMC 2019).

Complete this activity now

- Review the Future Nurse Standards of Proficiency (NMC 2018a).
- Identify two proficiencies that you have not achieved yet.
- Plan some CPD activities to help you to develop your knowledge and skills to achieve these proficiencies.

Practice-related feedback

Practice-related feedback can be obtained from people that you have looked after or colleagues you have worked with (NMC 2019). This element of the revalidation requirement seeks to embed practice related feedback into registrant's understanding of their own practice (NMC 2019). By doing this, it is hoped that registrants will become more responsive to the people who use their services and the teams they are working within (NMC 2019; Table 12.10).

TABLE 12.10

Practice-related feedback.

Requirement	Supporting evidence
Five pieces of practice-related feedback	• Notes on the content of the feedback and how you used it to improve your practice. This will be helpful for you to use when you are preparing your reflective accounts. • Make sure your notes do not include any personal data

Source: Adapted from NMC (2019).

Practice-related feedback can be obtained from many sources including service users, carers, students, colleagues, complaints, serious incident reviews and annual appraisal (NMC 2019). It can relate to an individual practitioner or to the wider team (NMC 2019). Practice-related feedback can be formal or informal and can be conveyed to practitioners in writing or verbally (NMC 2019). As a student you are likely to be familiar with practice-related feedback that you have received from your practice assessors; this requirement encourages you to think more broadly about where you can get feedback from.

Go online

The NMC has provided a useful template that is recommended to help registrants log their practice-related feedback. Practice-Related Feedback Log Template: www.nmc.org.uk/revalidation/resources/forms-and-templates

Seeking feedback from different people and varied sources adds depth and breadth to our own understanding of our everyday practice. This should help you to think about what you are already doing well and what elements of your practice may need further development. The NMC (2019) also encourages registrants to reflect carefully on any feedback received and consider how it relates to the Code (NMC 2018b). Please note that the professional obligations set out in standard 5 of the Code (NMC 2018b; Box 12.1) remain paramount when recording this feedback.

To reiterate, practice-related feedback must not include any information that might identify a service user, carer or colleague (NMC 2019). This means that any documentation should not include the person's name, the date of an incident or event, the location of an incident or event (e.g. ward name) or any unique information that could identify the person (NMC 2019). This kind of information should be removed or redacted from any practice-related feedback that you might obtain. This is to protect the person's identity and maintain confidentiality (NMC 2019). It is also vital that permission is sought to use information that belongs to an organisation or employer (NMC 2019) so if seeking feedback directly from service users, carers and colleagues, you should make it clear how you intend to use the feedback (NMC 2019). Service users should also be reassured that any feedback given will not affect the care they receive (NMC 2019).

Box 12.1 | Respect people's right to privacy and confidentiality

As a nurse, midwife or nursing associate, you owe a duty of confidentiality to all those who are receiving care. This includes making sure that they are informed about their care and that information about them is shared appropriately. To achieve this, you must:

5.1 Respect a person's right to privacy in all aspects of their care.

5.2 Make sure that people are informed about how and why information is used and shared by those who will be providing care.

5.3 Respect that a person's right to privacy and confidentiality continues after they have died.

5.4 Share necessary information with other health and care professionals and agencies only when the interests of patient safety and public protection override the need for confidentiality.

5.5 Share with people, their families and their carers, as far as the law allows, the information they want or need to know about their health, care and ongoing treatment sensitively and in a way they can understand.

Source: Adapted from NMC (2018).

It is important to not only obtain feedback but to consider the feedback, reflect on the positive aspects and the constructive development points and utilise that learning to improve future practice.

Written reflective accounts

Reflective practice is central to a nurse's professional identity. Reflection allows us to make sense of situations and identify areas for learning and development to include in CPD (NMC 2021b). The requirement for written reflective accounts hopes to embed reflection and reflective practice to enable practitioners to identify how to consolidate their good practices and pinpoint any elements of practice that might require attention or further development (NMC 2019). By reflecting on CPD, practice related feedback received and experiences and how they relate

TABLE **12.11**	

Reflective accounts.

Requirement	Supporting evidence
Five written reflective accounts	• Five written reflective accounts that explain what you learnt from your CPD activity and/or feedback and/or an event or experience in your practice, how you changed or improved your work as a result, and how this is relevant to the Code. • You must use the NMC form and make sure your accounts do not include any personal data.

Source: Adapted from NMC (2019).

to the four themes of the Code (prioritise people, practice effectively, preserve safety, promote professionalism and trust), it is anticipated that practitioners will have a more meaningful understanding of how the Code relates to their everyday practice and conduct (NMC 2019) (see Table 12.11).

Registrants can choose what they reflect upon which means that your reflection is meaningful to you and is allied to your own professional practice (NMC 2021b). Although these reflections will be discussed with your confirmer, there is freedom to reflect on both negative and positive situations so that worthwhile learning from reflection can be achieved (NMC 2019).

Go online

The NMC has provided the following form that is mandatory for registrants to log their reflective accounts (NMC 2019). These forms do not need to be submitted to the NMC but should be retained and used as the basis for a reflective discussion with your confirmer. Reflective Accounts Form: www.nmc.org.uk/revalidation/resources/forms-and-templates

There are numerous reflective models or processes that can support reflective activities (Thorpe 2022) however, the NMC (2021b) advocates that you should address the following questions when reflecting:

• What key things did you take away or learn from this experience/feedback?

- How did you address any issues or problems that arose?
- What would you do differently, if anything, next time around?
- How has it impacted on your practice?
- Are there any changes you can quickly apply to your practice?
- Are you able to support yourself and other colleagues better?
- What can you do to meet any gaps in your knowledge, skills and understanding?

Whichever way you choose to reflect on your practice, it is important that you use a consistent and structured approach to enable you to analyse and learn from your practice. This in turn will help to inform and improve the quality of the care you will deliver in future.

Over to you

Take some time out and choose some CPD, practice-related feedback or an event or experience from clinical placement to reflect upon. Once you have finished reflecting, complete the NMC reflective account form and consider how your reflection relates to the four themes of the Code.

Reflective discussion

This requirement mandates registrants to have a reflective discussion about their five written reflective accounts with another NMC registrant. During this discussion, the reflective accounts will be considered in relation to the Code (NMC 2018a,b). This reflective discussion requires a sound understanding of the Code. It may be helpful to have a copy of the Code with you when having this discussion (NMC 2019). This aspect of revalidation aims to ensure that practitioners share their ideas about their own development and how clinical practice can be developed or improved. This culture of sharing, reflection and continual improvement should in turn help to reduce professional isolation and promote lifelong learning based on lived experiences (NMC 2019; Table 12.12).

It is worth giving some thought to who you would like to hold this reflective discussion with. Registrants have often used their line manager to have this conversation but this is not stipulated by the NMC (2019). Indeed, they encourage you to choose the 'most appropriate person;' it does not matter if they are at a higher or lower grade than yourself (NMC 2019, p. 29) although you may wish to consider a senior colleague if you feel they may be better suited to help support the reflective discussion.

> **TABLE 12.12**
>
> **Practice related feedback.**
>
> | Requirement | Supporting evidence |
> | --- | --- |
> | Reflective discussion | • A reflective discussion form which includes the name and NMC Pin of the NMC-registered nurse, midwife or nursing associate that you had the discussion with as well as the date you had the discussion.
• You must use the NMC form and make sure the discussion summary section does not contain any personal data |
>
> *Source:* Adapted from NMC (2019).

The NMC (2019, p. 29) sets out the following guidance on who should be your reflective discussion partner:

- They must be a nurse, midwife or nursing associate with an effective registration with the NMC, by which they cannot be subject to any kind of suspension, removal or striking-off order at the time of having the discussion.
- They could be someone you frequently work with or someone from a professional network or learning group.
- They do not need to be someone you work with on a daily basis.
- They do not need to undertake the same type of practice as you.
- They do not need to be on the same part of the register as you (so a nurse can have a reflective discussion with a midwife and vice versa).

The advantage of this approach is that it encourages practitioners who do not work in a setting with other registrants to find people within professional or specialty-based networks with whom to hold these discussions and in doing so, also reduce potential professional isolation (NMC 2019).

Go online

The NMC has provided the following form that is mandatory for registrants to log their reflective discussion (NMC 2019). These forms do not need to be submitted to the NMC but should be retained and used as the basis for a reflective discussion with your confirmer. Reflective Discussion Form: www.nmc.org.uk/revalidation/resources/forms-and-templates

This reflective discussion is only required once every three years when the registrant's revalidation is due but the NMC (2021b) encourages practitioners to use reflection and reflective discussion as part of everyday practice and lifelong learning. These discussions can take place in a variety of formats such as reflective practice groups, case reviews or debriefs. By doing this, practitioners embed cycles of positive and meaningful service improvements that are rooted in supportive and reflective activities with other healthcare professionals (NMC 2021b).

Over to you

Building on the previous reflective activity, sit down with one of your peers or a practice supervisor/assessor and hold a reflective discussion based on your reflective account. Make sure that you have a copy of the Code (NMC 2018b) with you. Think about how you can use this conversation to identify what you need to do next in terms of your CPD and how you will use learning prompted by this discussion to inform and improve the care you deliver.

Additional requirements for revalidation

There are some additional elements that are required by the NMC to complete your triennial (three-yearly) revalidation:

- A declaration of your health and character is required to assure the NMC that you are still able to provide safe care for our patients and service users.
- Evidence of professional indemnity arrangements must also be provided. This measure should assure the public that if they suffer any harm resulting from the negligent activity of someone on the register, they will receive the appropriate compensation (NMC 2021g).
- Finally, the NMC (2019) requires that all the elements of revalidation are verified by an appropriate confirmer who will provide their professional details to the NMC when you submit your application to revalidate. See Table 12.13 for these additional requirements.

	TABLE **12.13**

Additional requirements.

Requirement	Supporting evidence
Health and character	• You must make a declaration as to your health and character as part of your online revalidation application.
Professional indemnity arrangement	• Evidence to demonstrate that you have an appropriate indemnity arrangement in place. • You must tell us whether your indemnity arrangement is through your employer, membership of a professional body or through a private insurance arrangement. • If your indemnity arrangement is provided through membership of a professional body or a private insurance arrangement, you will need to record the name of the professional body or provider.
Confirmation	• A confirmation form signed by confirmer.

Source: Adapted from NMC (2019).

Go online

Examples of completed revalidation forms and templates are available from the NMC: https://www.nmc.org.uk/revalidation/resources/forms-and-templates

If you need some inspiration these forms can be a useful place to start!

Summary

This chapter has considered the importance of lifelong learning to you, your employer, the people you have the privilege to care for and the wider system once you have joined the professional register. The principles of lifelong learning are embedded into the NMC (2019) revalidation processes. To maintain your professional registration, it is important that you have a good understanding of what is required and the many opportunities you will have to meet these requirements.

References

Francis, R. (2013). *Report of the Mid Staffordshire NHS Foundation Trust Public Inquiry*. HC 898-III. London: Stationery Office https://assets.publishing.service.gov.uk/government/uploads/system/uploads/attachment_data/file/279124/0947.pdf (accessed 4 June 2022).

Interprofessional CPD and Lifelong Learning UK Working Group (2019) *Principles for Continuing Professional Development and Lifelong Learning in Health and Social Care*. Bridgwater: College of Paramedics. https://collegeofparamedics.co.uk/COP/[COP]/Professional_development/Principles_for_CPD/COP/ProfessionalDevelopment/Principles_for_CPD.aspx?hkey=c1310302-0b10-41cc-b071-5b1caf876f01 (accessed 30 May 2022).

Nursing and Midwifery Council (2018a). *Future Nurse: The Standards of Proficiency for Registered Nurses*. www.nmc.org.uk/globalassets/sitedocuments/education-standards/future-nurse-proficiencies.pdf (accessed 20 March 2023).

Nursing and Midwifery Council (2018b) *The Code: Professional Standards of Practice and Behaviour for Nurses, Midwives and Nursing Associates*. www.nmc.org.uk/standards/code (accessed 5 June 2022).

Nursing and Midwifery Council (2019) *Revalidation: How to revalidate with the NMC*. London: NMC.

Nursing and Midwifery Council (2021a) *Continuing professional development. Guidance Sheet – Examples of CPD activities*. London: NMC. https://www.nmc.org.uk/revalidation/requirements/cpd (accessed 3 June 2022).

Nursing and Midwifery Council (2021b) *Reflective Practice. Guidance Sheet*. London: NMC. www.nmc.org.uk/revalidation/requirements/reflective-discussion (accessed 26 April 2022).

Thorpe, G. (2022). Reflection and evidence based practice. In: *Essentials of Nursing Practice*, 3e (ed. C. Delves-Yates), 37–55. London: Sage.

INDEX

Page locators in *italics* indicate figures. This index uses letter-by-letter alphabetization.

Succeeding on your Nursing Placement: Supervision, Learning and Assessment for Nursing Students, First Edition. Edited by Ian Peate.
© 2024 John Wiley & Sons Ltd. Published 2024 by John Wiley & Sons Ltd.